YOGI ON THE GREEN

By Victor Stringer

Published by Best Seller Publishing®, Pasadena, CA
Best Seller Publishing® is a registered trademark
Printed in the United States of America.
ISBN 978-1-946978-29-5

This publication is designed to provide accurate and authoritative information with regard to the subject matter covered. It is sold with the understanding that the publisher is not engaged in rendering legal, accounting, or other professional advice. If legal advice or other expert assistance is required, the services of a competent professional should be sought. The opinions expressed by the authors in this book are not endorsed by Best Seller Publishing® and are the sole responsibility of the author rendering the opinion.

Most Best Seller Publishing® titles are available at special quantity discounts for bulk purchases for sales promotions, premiums, fundraising, and educational use. Special versions or book excerpts can also be created to fit specific needs.

For more information, please write:
Best Seller Publishing®
1346 Walnut Street, #205
Pasadena, CA 91106
or call 1(626) 765 9750
Toll Free: 1(844) 850-3500
Visit us online at: www.BestSellerPublishing.org

TABLE OF CONTENTS

INTRODUCTION

In the first part of 2001, my business took a down turn and I lost many clients. Everything was very difficult for me at that time, and I felt lost in every aspect of my life. I had no focus.

A friend of mine who was teaching yoga suggested I might give it a try. I knew very little about yoga and was somewhat skeptical, but what could be the harm in trying? So, I attended a few classes, and to my surprise, I was soon hooked. But it wasn't only the classes themselves I enjoyed. I found that I could apply the techniques I learned in the classes to my everyday activities and, in doing so, my attitude towards the rest of my life began to change; it became more positive, and I became more relaxed. During this difficult time, that feeling was wonderful.

After a few months of taking the classes, I enrolled in a training course for Kundalini yoga teachers in Los Angeles. The course was taught by Yogi Bhajan, the guru who introduced Kundalini yoga to the United States in the 1970s. From this point, my life seemed to improve even more. My business recovered, and my personal life had greater meaning because there was less stress. Yoga helped me take control of the things I could do something about and let go of the things I could not control, or at least stop them controlling me.

Overall, I would have to say that yoga has given me a better outlook on life. I am less stressed, more focused, and in better condition, both physically and mentally, than at any other time in my life.

But what about golf? I took up golf around the age of 40. Prior to that, I had played all forms of sports: tennis, football, Judo, baseball, cycling . . . you name it, I tried it! Nothing gave me a better sense of self than golf because it is a solitary game, even if you're playing in a group. It was the only sport I could play and be focused on myself. I could practice—every day if I wanted to—without needing someone else to play with. Being outdoors, rain or shine, was also the attraction. Golf is a game that allows you to enjoy some spectacular scenery, and I play in all conditions.

After only three months of playing the game, I got a hole-in-one, but it was an experience I would not have again for another 20 years. I became a good golfer—with a solid 10 handicap—but I wasn't the golfer I wanted to be. It seemed that no matter how committed I was to improving, I wasn't able to better a 70 score. There always seemed to be one shot that ruined my entire round.

I didn't take lessons for over 10 years. When I finally took one, it only made my game worse! I spent a lot of money on the latest high-tech equipment, but nothing helped. I was spending more money on equipment than I was spending to play the game. Then a friend told me, "Sometimes the problem is the archer, not the arrow." It was then I realized the problem was not my swing or my clubs: it was me. I am sure every golfer has this revelation at some point.

It wasn't until I took up yoga that I experienced an improvement in my game. I'll explain later in the book, but for now I'll simply say that yoga helped me reduce my handicap from 10 to 3. I won a lot of tournaments and long-drive contests (for which I always received a new driver!).

During one of my yoga classes, I thought about how yoga helped me improve my golf game, and it finally dawned on me that perhaps, I could help other golfers improve their games and that yoga could even help players enhance other areas of their life, too.

The great American golfer Arnold Palmer once said: "I have a tip that can take five strokes off anyone's game; it's called an eraser." Through this book, I will introduce a way to better your game in a more honest and healthy way: yoga.

There are many books about yoga and perhaps just as many about golf, so it is not my intention to go into great detail about either discipline. This book is simply for the golfer who is keen to try any means of enhancing his or her game and curious about trying yoga. I have attempted to give you an overview of the subjects in the hope that you will seek out professionals that will help you become as proficient as you desire. It is important that you create a training program for yourself that helps make you the golfer you want to be and the person you desire to see in the mirror every morning.

It is my wish that this humble book inspires you explore the benefits of yoga on your game, and I sincerely hope you go on to become a yogi, not only on the fairway and the green, but also in the sand trap and the rough and may the practice of Yoga also, help you to improve all aspects of your life as well.

Chapter 1

YOGA 101

Yoga is a hugely popular form of exercise all over the United States, especially in California, where I live. Wherever you live, I expect you'll have seen a lot of people in Lycra carrying rolled-up mats on their way to the gym. But yoga is not a modern "exercise fad."

A Brief History of Yoga

Yoga originated in South Asia many centuries ago. In the 1920s, noted archaeologist Sir John Hubert Marshall was heading a mission to uncover the long-gone civilizations of the Indus Valley and excavated ancient Buddhist sculptures, artwork, and figurines depicting people in various postures. The artefacts were dated between 2500 B.C. and 1750 A.D. These days we often associate yoga with Hinduism, but it probably began with Buddhism, and some researchers believe that the roots of yoga can be traced back to Shamanism as far as 25,000 B.C., so yoga probably has a very long history indeed.

Practitioners of yoga are called "yogis," and they are similar to shamans in their quest for enlightenment. But what is enlightenment? This was a question once asked of Buddha by a follower. So the story goes, the Buddha answered the student's question with a question of his own: "Are you aware that you are standing?" The student (no doubt confused by the question) replied yes, to which the Buddha replied, "Then you are enlightened." What the Buddha was suggesting is that yoga is as much an intellectual practice as it is a physical exercise.

In fact, the word yoga derives from the word "yoke," meaning to bind together. The things being bound in yoga are the body and the mind. In the beginning, yoga was more focused on giving people the mental strength to deal with life's hardships and transcending their physical incarnation. These days, the focus of yoga is almost completely on the body. One of the reasons yoga was not introduced to the U.S. before the 1900s is that yoga masters did not want their teachings turned into an exercise program; of course, yoga is now considered by many Westerners to be just that, and these days, the practice of yoga—for most people—has very little to do with its religious and cultural roots.

Forms of Yoga

Yoga is a very general term. To understand it properly, think of yoga as a river with six tributaries, each flowing with a different energy.

Raja – Meditation
> Also known as "Royal Yoga" because practitioners become rulers of their mind.

Hatha – Force
> Practitioners build physical and mental strength.

Karma – Selflessness
> A practice that seeks to atone for your previous selfish deeds in this life and includes service to others.

Bhakti – Heart (Devotion)
> The most religious branch of yoga, commonly practiced in India in worship of the Hindu deity Krishna. It can include rites and songs. In the West, it is about connecting with and surrendering to the Divine.

Jnana – Wisdom

Perhaps the most "conscious" of all the yoga forms, Jnana is all about achieving oneness with all life. It involves a lot of introspection and a mastery of the mind.

Tantra – Sacred Ritual

A highly meditative, focused form of yoga that works on your energy centers (known as chakras). In the West, the word "tantric" is often associated with sex, but this kind of yoga is really about strength, clarity, and bliss.

Hatha is the umbrella term for several forms of the more physical yoga practices—the kind of yoga you would find on a gym's class schedule. Hatha yoga binds body and mind through postures known as asanas.

The earliest descriptions of asanas are to be found in the text *Hatha Yoga Pradipika*, written in the fourteenth century, which names 15 asana postures. Asana is a Sanskrit word meaning chair or seat. In the same way that one sits for periods of time in varying positions on a chair, yogis hold various poses (asanas) for seconds, minutes, and sometimes hours. Many of the asanas we know today may have been developed as late at the nineteenth century.

Hatha yoga is going to be the focus of this book, and we'll go into the specific poses that are featured in hatha yoga in later chapters. I trained in Kundalini yoga, but you may want to try others, which I have outlined below. Of course, which one you choose to try will probably be determined by what's available in your area.

Kundalini.

This is the form of yoga I trained in. Kundalini involves movement, breathing, and meditation, and it's one of the most popular forms of yoga. I'm told that the word means "the curl of the lock of hair of the beloved." This poetic definition is said to reflect the flow of energy (body) and consciousness (mind) that are merged during yoga practice.

Ashtanga.

This form of yoga is one of the most physical, and it emphasizes breathing and movement through "vinyasas," which are the movements between poses. Vinyasas link asanas together in set-piece sequences. Because there's a lot of movement, it's good for core strength and muscle toning.

Iyengar.

This form of yoga is all about precision. It focuses on parts of the body and can involve holding poses for longer periods, often with the use of props (blocks, belts, chairs, etc.). It is great for developing balance, strength, and focus.

Acro.

A sociable form of yoga practiced in pairs with a partner.

Bikram (hot yoga).

A version of yoga designed to make you sweat. The room is kept warm and the yoga is more physical. Heat makes your muscles and tendons more pliable.

Upa Yoga.

This form has no spiritual aspect and takes less time to perform (as little as 20 minutes). Known as "pre-yoga" or "sub-yoga," Upa offers simple yet powerful sets of 10 practices designed to lubricate the joints and activate the energy system and muscles, which bring ease to the whole body.

Many forms of yoga involve "props"—accessories for helping you during a class. A gym will often have what you need for a yoga class, but most people prefer to use their own props.

1. Yoga is done barefoot, so a **mat** helps you maintain your grip on the hard floor and provides some cushion to protect your knees, elbows, etc.

2. Yoga involves a lot of stretching, and a **strap** or **belt** can help people who are less flexible get into and maintain poses.
3. A soft **block** or **brick** provides three heights for the beginner yogi who needs help reaching the floor or some balance support. It is wise to own two—one for each hand.
4. A **bolster** is a long, somewhat flat pillow that is sat upon to give some height in sitting poses or support for the back during floor exercises.
5. Like the bolster, the **blanket** can be folded and used for sitting poses. It is also used to provide some warmth during the relaxation part of the yoga class.

Benefits of Yoga

The writer Malcolm Gladwell, in his book *Outliers*, famously claimed that it takes 10,000 hours to become proficient in anything. That's three hours per day for ten years! I don't expect you can practice yoga that much, but it will take some time to see the effects on your body and mind, so a regular practice is essential. Even the yoga masters talk about yoga in terms of "practice" because it is something one is continuously trying to perfect—like the amateur and his golf game!

I referred in the introduction to the positivity that yoga brought back into my life during a difficult period, and you may have wondered how a few stretches and some meditation can create a positive life change. It is well known that physical exercise can improve our mental health. Of course, people feel better about themselves when they see the impact exercise has on their waistline, but regular workouts also release serotonin (the so-called happy hormone). This is true of yoga, too, but yoga can offer something that the treadmill cannot: peace of mind and focus.

The meditative, relaxation aspects of yoga encourage us to clear our minds, which is not something we usually have much time for in our busy lives. When was the last time you consciously switched off your overworked brain for even a minute? Yoga also encourages us to focus on how we feel in our bodies and minds, and there is something both uplifting and healing about self-reflection. That is my experience, at least. But what else can yoga do for you?

Stronger muscles. The asanas build and condition your muscles.

Greater flexibility. Stretching exercises improves elasticity in all the ligaments and muscles for a greater range of movement.

Improved posture. Yoga's focus on healthy body positioning reduces muscle strain and neck and back problems.

Protects joints and vertebrae. By putting the body through a full range of motion, yoga releases nutrients to the joints and spine, keeping them supple.

Stronger bones. Exercises in which you are supporting your own weight improves bone density.

Cardiovascular conditioning. Yoga is a gentle way to raise the heart rate. Some of the "inversions" (upside-down poses or lying-down postures where your legs are lifted) also give your heart a well-earned rest.

Oxygen flow. The aerobic exercise combined with the breathing in yoga increases the flow of oxygen in the blood to your organs, heart, and brain.

Increased oxygen to the brain can improve cognitive function. Deeper breathing also improves your lung capacity.

Reduces hypertension. The relaxation involved in yoga also lowers blood pressure (by lowering the stress hormone cortisol). And when we are less stressed, we sleep better.

Boosts immunity. The movements in yoga help drain your lymph nodes, releasing more immunity cells.

Improves balance. Through the various balance postures, we train our bodies to be more stable.

Better digestion. Several asanas provide interior massage, which can benefit our digestive tract.

Improve athletic performance.

All of the above benefits combine to help protect you from injury.

I trained as a Kundalini yoga instructor in 2001. At my first class, I had the pleasure of meeting Shakri Parwha Khalsa, one of the most inspiring people I've ever met. At the time, she had been teaching for over 25 years. Her straight talk, simple-to-understand directions, and her smile made all the classes enjoyable.

Studying and teaching yoga has given me new ideas, new ways of looking at myself and the others in my life, and new ways to deal with every aspect of my life. I am able to live my life on a higher level of consciousness thanks to Kundalini yoga.

There are many paths a person can take to their future and yoga helped me keep to the path I chose and to have faith that I will stay on that path going forward.

I hope I have made it clear what you stand to gain from exploring yoga. In the next chapter, my aim is to persuade you to see the benefits of doing so for the sake of your golf game and your life.

Chapter 2

YOGA AND
YOUR GAME

On a trivial level, yoga and golf have one thing in common: their affinity with animals. Many asanas have English names such as cobra, downward dog, pigeon, and crow. Similarly, golfing vocabulary includes dog leg, eagle, albatross, and rabbit. But there is so much more to the relationship between the two disciplines than the animal vocabulary.

Before I get into what yoga can do for your golf game, I want to start with a fun history of the game we know and love.

A Brief History of Golf

> *"Golf is not a matter of life or death: It is much more important than that."*
> —Unknown

There are thought to be more than 34,000 golf courses around the world, and more than half of those are in the United States. Golf is played by millions of people worldwide, people of all ages and from all walks of life—some are serious professional players, some are fair-weather hobbyists. These days, golf is a multibillion-dollar industry, but it has very humble origins.

Golf is most associated with Scotland, and legend has it that the game began as a walking sport in the fifteenth century. Sailors on shore leave near the city of St. Andrews would use sticks to hit rocks as far as they could, and informal contests soon emerged. At first, the game was to hit the rock the farthest. Then it became a game of accuracy; a contest of who could get nearest a target. This is a romantic story, and there are some that would disagree on the true origin of golf. Some historians believe the game was invented by the Dutch a century before it was believed to have begun in Scotland. And other historians trace the game back to China during the Song dynasty (960 to 1279).

Wherever it began, it is true that the oldest golf course in the world is the Royal Blackheath Golf Club. According to W.E. Hughes, author of *Chronicles of Blackheath Golfers* (1897), the club began in 1608 and was granted Royal patronage by King James I, although written records for the club did not begin until 1787. Playing this course is on my bucket list.

India was one of the first places outside the British Isles to embrace the sport, and the first club in India—the Royal Calcutta Golf Club—formed in 1829. This is the oldest club outside of Great Britain and, at the time of writing, it is still ranked in the top 10 of the world's 100 best golf courses.

The longest course in the world is said to be the Jade Dragon Snow Mountain Golf Club in the Chinese Himalayas. It is a total of 8548 yards and a par 72. At an altitude of 10,800 feet, it is also the highest golf course and oxygen tanks are provided with the golf cart! But there is also the Nullarbor Links in southern Australia, a par 73 course that stretches over 1365 kilometers along the Eyre Highway.

The longest holes are a par 7,949-yard fairway at the Sutsuki Golf Course in Japan, and a 1007-yard, par 6, double-dogleg fairway at the Chocoloy Downs course in the U.S. state of Michigan.

The longest Par 3 hold in the world is the 19th Hole at the Legends Golf Course, South Africa. The hole is nearly 400 yards long and the Tee is on top of a Mountain some 400 meters above the hold and is only accessible by Helicopter. The first person to par the hole, was PGA Professions Padraig Harrington.

And finally, I've heard that the origin of the term "caddie" is attributed to Mary Queen of Scots. She was educated in France where she engaged a French cadet to carry her clubs. The Scottish spelling of "caddie" comes from the French pronunciation of "cadet."

Health Benefits and Risks of Golf

"Bask in the sun; spend time in the open air. The sun and the open air are your good doctor. Take sufficient exercise, become your own physician."
—The Yoga Cookbook: Vegetarian Food for Body and Mind
(by Sivananda Yoga Vedanta Center)

Because golf is often taken up by retirees, people who play might not consider themselves *athletes*. Most top professional players are all at a peak of physical fitness; nevertheless, most employ a personal trainer as part of their quest for success. Amateurs too—regardless of age—should aim to be as fit as possible if their game is going to improve.

The exercise you get from playing golf is an obvious benefit. Walking considerable distances carrying (or pulling on a trolley) a bag full of clubs can help you lose weight as well as build muscle and bone density. During a game, a golfer might take as many as 20,000 steps, but if you drive a cart everywhere, the physical benefits are going to be much less clear. I once played golf with a gentleman in his 80s who told me he played every single day and claimed golf was what kept him alive. There may be a scientific reason for his claim because some researchers have reported that those who play golf live five years longer on average than people who do not.

In September 2016, researchers at the University of Aberdeen, Scotland, published a piece in the *British Journal of Sports Medicine* about the health benefits of golf. The researchers collected more than 5,000 studies and concluded that the game is particularly good for heart health because of the increased blood flow. There were also proven benefits to mental health, cognition, weight control, blood pressure, balance, and bone density. A round of golf can also give you a better night's sleep.

Golf is good for the brain, too. Doctor Clive Ballard, director of research at the Alzheimer's Society in the United Kingdom from 2003 to 2013, said: "Whether it's going for a jog or walking the golf course, keeping physically active is a great way to give your brain a good, strong blood supply, which is essential to its function now and in the future."

There is also something I call the D Factor. Being out in the sunshine is a great way to boost your vitamin D, which is proven to lower blood sugar levels and improve one's mood, and some research even suggests that vitamin D may reduce the risk of some cancers and improve your immune system. Golf is good for your mood, too. Even when the game is frustrating, exercising outside in the fresh air, often in beautiful scenery, has obvious advantages. The highly sociable nature of golf (especially at the 19th hole) also helps us to feel good. And think of the business benefits—how many deals have been made on the fairway?

But unless your body is properly conditioned, playing golf can do you more harm than good. Many golfers will experience an injury at one time or another—even the professionals with their personal trainers! According to Doctor Jeffrey H. Blanchard, golf professional and a doctor of chiropractic medicine, 30 percent of all professional golfers are playing injured (54 percent of those are male golfers and 43 percent are female). Those injuries might be one of the following.

Lower back stress.

Practicing your swing for hours can put undue stress on your lower back muscles. The great Tiger Woods suffered from this problem, and he lost several tournaments and missed many others as a result.

Tennis elbow.

This painful condition is an inflammation of the outer tendon of the elbow.

Golfer elbow.

This is an inflammation of the inner tendon, which causes a great deal of discomfort.

Knee injury.

You can damage your knees if your hips do not rotate correctly during your swing. This is a problem for older golfers whose joints might be deteriorating naturally with age.

Tendonitis.

The wrists play a big role in your swing and golfers can suffer from inflammation of the tendons in the wrist joint.

Rotator cuff injury.

Golf can take its toll on your shoulders too. Sometimes serious damage is caused by hitting the ground hard during a poor swing.

Hand injuries.

These can be sustained if you have a poor grip.

Neck injury.

Common among novice golfers who aren't used to twisting their bodies and may not keep their head still during their swing.

Hip injury.

The hips do a lot of work during the swing. The joint is similar to your shoulder's rotator cuff, so it is also prone to the same damage.

Sunburn.

This is not a widely acknowledged risk of golf. Some sunshine is good for the vitamin D levels, but don't succumb to sunstroke or put yourself at risk of skin cancer.

With the exception of sunburn, yoga can help you minimize the risk of all these injuries through the benefits yoga has on your joints, flexibility, and strength. Also, because golfers tend to favor one side (even the professional golfer Phil Michelson who is right-handed but plays from his left side), yoga is a great way to help us develop a better physical balance in our bodies. The practice of yoga balances all the muscles' movements, right and left; every movement is symmetrical.

Yoga is a particularly good option for people who feel they cannot do "high-impact" fitness training—such as running, cycling, or weights—to get fitter, and we'll explore the best asanas for your game in chapters three through five.

But yoga also has less obvious advantages for the golfer, benefits that are not physical but mental.

Golf: A Game of Mental Strength

"Ninety percent of golf is played from the shoulders up."
—Deacon Palmer, father of US pro golfer Arnold Palmer

There is a reason why touring golfers often travel with a fitness trainer *and* a sports psychologist. On difficult days, golf is referred to as "flog" (golf spelled backwards) because it can take its toll on the body and mind.

In order to play golf well, the game demands that the body and the mind be in perfect union. The body must be fit enough to power the ball, and at the same time, the mind must focus on every element of the swing, which include:

Target line
Plane line
Vertical plane
Horizontal plane
Incline plane
Swing plane
Pivot
Loading

Set Point
Unloading

As you can see, there are a lot of things going on in a golfer's mind when he or she is getting ready to swing, so it's important not to be distracted.

When body and mind are in harmony, some golfers say they are in "the zone." This is probably what Mary "Mickey" Wright meant when she said: "When I play my best golf, I feel as if I'm in a fog, standing back watching Earth in orbit with a golf club in my hands."

When you are in the zone, there is no better feeling than to see the ball land at the intended place; when you're not in the zone, failure to strike the ball can severely damage self-confidence. We can't all be as sure of ourselves as the Puerto Rican champion Chi Chi Rodriquez, who once said, "I'm gonna be a firecracker out there today. I'm gonna be so hot, they're gonna be playing on brown fairways tomorrow!"

In his book, *If You Play Golf, You're My Friend*, the great American player Harvey Penick describes an experience he had coaching professional golfer Barbara Puett, who went to Penick for advice, frustrated that no matter how she adjusted her swing, she kept hitting behind the ball. Penick assessed her swing and then sent her home to practice hitting one spot regularly with a 7 iron. He told her that until she could do that perfectly, there was nothing he could do for her.

Sometime later, Penick saw Puett at a LPGA event and was impressed by her score. He asked her what had changed, and she told him that she had realized she couldn't hit the spot because her mind wasn't on it. "Once I quit thinking about my swing," she said, "and put my mind to hitting the spot instead, the problem went away." If a top professional like Barbara Puett had trouble focusing her mind on the right things, amateurs are surely going to struggle!

As the professional player Sam Snead said: "Thinking instead of acting is the number one golf disease." The quality of the expensive clubs in your bag will mean very little if your mental approach to the game is unfocused. It's all about keeping your concentration and keeping calm. As the Buddha once said, "As you think, so your world becomes."

Concentration, like most things in life, requires practice. It only takes a split second to be distracted, and there are plenty of potential distractions both on the golf course and in your own mind. Distractions are the golfer's downfall. I have seen many a professional golfer put off their games by someone in the crowd with a camera. At that point, the player must begin the pre-shot routine all over again and hope the damage hasn't been done.

For many amateurs, there can be very little etiquette on the fairway, especially if you're playing a casual game with friends. Ben Hogan once said, "I play with friends, but we don't play friendly games." So, if you want your game to improve, you have to stop your friends becoming a distraction. I used to play golf with a guy who talked the entire time, even when other players in the group were attempting to set up their tee shots. On occasion, when he distracted me, I would stand back from the tee and wait. When he asked me if I was going to hit the ball, I replied, "I don't want to interrupt your conversation!" I really enjoyed hanging out with him off the course; however, when he told me he was joining another club, I was happy. After that, my game didn't improve much, but I got greater enjoyment from playing.

It also takes mental toughness to learn from your mistakes, rather than let the mistakes defeat you. Pro golfer Paul Azinger put it like this: "Great champions learn from past experiences, whether those experiences be bad good or bad. A lot of times, a guy needs to be knocked down before he gets up and fights."

Overall, then, it's safe to say that golfers who see the game as purely physical are making a big mistake. The emphasis on mindfulness in yoga teaches us how to stay in the moment and not stress over things that are out of your control, and the meditative aspects to yoga help us manage emotions, focus, and relax: A calmer player leads to a better game. (We'll return to the issue of mindfulness in chapter six.)

My aim in the first two chapters was to persuade you of the many benefits to working yoga into your golfing life, and I recommend going to yoga classes as often as you go to the practice range. But if you're still wondering whether yoga can really help you, it is worth pointing out that the practice of yoga is frequently used by athletes in a range of sports.

Football

The Seattle Seahawks were so impressed by the benefits of yoga that they introduced an optional yoga program, which was then made mandatory. The team members can participate in a meditation program.

Baseball

Evan Longoria, third baseman of the Tampa Bay Rays, practices yoga. He says, "When you're hitting, you want to be as stable as you can and use the three-dimensional aspect—the rotation of your core—to actually translate to power."

Basketball

Blake Griffin of the LA Clippers enjoys the flexibility yoga gives him, which he uses to stay loose on the court. He even adapted various yoga poses using a basketball.[1]

Cricket

South Asia is the birthplace of yoga, so it's no surprise that Indian and Pakistani cricketers limber up for the game with yoga moves. The skill of focusing the mind in yoga is also thought to help players connect the bat with the ball and relieve stress during the game.

---

1   http://www.mensfitness.com/training/combine-basketball-and-yoga-moves

Track

Runners are increasingly turning to yoga because it is a great way to ensure bodily symmetry and awareness. A poor posture and uneven running style can cause runners injury. Yoga also helps in post-race recovery.

Many sportspeople have embraced yoga and seen the benefits, so perhaps it's time you did too! But it is important to remember we are all at different places with our strength and flexibility. If you happen to be concerned about going for yoga instruction, it is okay to use this book to help you practice some basic yoga poses at home until you wish to expand your abilities and are more confident in seeking a yoga instructor. Yogi Bhajan, in his book *The Master's Touch*, says that "When you are ready for a teacher, a teacher is ready for you." I have heard this expression many times over the past 30 years and know it to be true.

Yoga will not improve your golf game overnight because nothing can! I remember reading that Nick Faldo, who had already won countless tournaments, was experiencing problems with his golf swing. He went to a teaching pro (whom I believe was David Ledbetter), and as the story goes, Ledbetter informed Faldo that he knew what the problem was, but it would take two years to fix. Two years! This did not fit well with Faldo's plans, so he tried to fix the problem himself. He failed and returned to Ledbetter for help. Almost two years later, the problem was solved and Faldo returned to the PGA Tour and won several more major tournaments over the next few years. The point is to take your time, relax, and practice: All that you seek will eventually come to you.

Words of Advice for the Yoga Beginner

In the next few chapters, I'm going to introduce you to the poses that will help condition your body and mind and improve your game. In the meantime, however, here are some things to keep in mind.

1. Many of the asanas look very straightforward; nevertheless, I do not recommend trying them for the first time without the guidance from a qualified yoga instructor. Yoga may be low impact, but it is still possible to injure yourself quite badly if you get a pose wrong. Once you have had a number of lessons with a professional and feel more confident to practice by yourself, use the forthcoming chapters to guide your regular yoga exercise at home.

2. You should also remember that whatever you do with the right side of your body, you should do with your left. This ensures balance. Do this even though it will be difficult. Because we favor either the left or right sides of our bodies, our muscles and ability to balance will be different on each side at first.

3. Women who are pregnant should seek a specialist yoga class because there are some poses that should not be attempted while pregnant.

4. Current or former joint injuries, carpal tunnel syndrome, or high blood pressure can also be considerations for your yoga practice. You should always inform the yoga instructor about specific health issues (or seek specialist advice) before taking the class. A good yoga instructor will be able to find adaptations for each pose that will take your injury or condition into account.

5. Do you know the phrase "No pain, no gain"? Well, in yoga, this does not apply. Yoga poses should be challenging, but they should not be painful (except the burn of lactic acid in your muscles). Yoga teachers encourage you to listen to your body, and if something is hurting, come out of the pose as gently as possible.

6. I once read that it takes at least 40 days to establish a habit, 90 days to confirm the habit, and 120 days to see the difference. Just as beginning to play golf is a matter of learning and developing good habits, the practice of yoga requires some patience and commitment. Habitual movements will create muscle memory.

7. Yoga is like most other activities that you learn during your life: You get more out of it the more you put into it. I am reminded about a story I heard years ago about at young American minister traveling through the South, who stopped by a small church on one Sunday morning. On a table by the door of the church there was a box for donations, and the young minister put in five dollars. As he was leaving, he paid his respects to the church's minster. The minister, who earlier had seen the younger man make his donation, opened the box and returned the money to him. The young minster said, "But there is just a five-dollar bill in the box!" to which the older minister, replied, "Well, the more you put in, the more you can get out."

8. When you are practicing golf or yoga, do not listen to that inner voice saying, "You can't do this!" You must learn to distinguish between discomfort and pain. If you are in pain, stop at once, relax, and try something else. If you experience difficulty, keep pushing forward: The reward is the doing. And remember that thinking you can't do something is the surest way not to do anything! You are much stronger than you might think.

Over the years, I have found that I perform better because I am more flexible, my range of motion has increased. Working on muscles in my chest, lateral muscles, and hips flexors, I attained greater flexibility by elongating the time I held stretches, which lengthened my muscles and the tendons around the bones that can tighten during normal daily activities.

Part of my daily workout includes squats, push-ups, lunges, side lunges, jumping jacks, and both sitting and standing twists. I also work on the core muscles. I tend to hold these stretches between 5 and 15 minutes each, doing several repetitions on each side of my body. Some of the postures (asanas) can be held up to 30 minutes. It is also important to change your workout daily; by doing so you improve on your entire body and your health.

But before I do my daily workout, I spend about 10 minutes just relaxing and breathing. By doing so I infuse more oxygen into my body, which helps me warm up my body, which in turn helps prevent injury. These postures are very much a part of my daily meditation (more on that topic in chapter six).

I hope the information contained in the coming chapters help you develop a regular exercise and meditation practice that will improve your golf game beyond your wildest expectations.

Chapter 3

WARM-UP &
STRETCHING

All good athletes know how important stretching is before exerting the body in any way. Golf may be a gentler sport than most, but stretching is still very important; your muscles must be ready to play.

For the most part, golfers have a tendency to get out of their cars, put on their golf shoes, and immediately start hitting the balls as far as they can. This shocks the body and the shock remains for the entire game. By taking only 10 minutes to warm up, you will do your body a lot of good. The energy released through stretching will also give you more energy for the game.

By using a good stretch routine, golfers will also increase the range of movement in their joints that will help extend their swing, which in turn will inject more power into the drive. Proper stretching will help reduce the number and severity of injuries, too.

Before we go on, however, I want to give one important instruction: **During your game and exercise, including warm-up, make sure you are well hydrated!** Not enough attention is paid to this part of your game and your workout program, which is unfortunate because being properly hydrated has a major impact on your flexibility and on your muscles' ability to perform well. Research shows that the brain and heart are 73 percent water, the lungs about 83 percent, the skin about 64 percent, and the muscles and kidneys about 79 percent. Even bones are about 31 percent water.[2] Water is better than sugary energy drinks.

---

2   H.H. Mitchell, *Journal of Biological Chemistry*, December 2, 2016.

Another benefit of water after a workout is that the water can flush out the waste products in your body that can impede your training.

So, grab your water bottle and let's get warm!

Shoulder Shrugs

- In a standing position, feet shoulder-width apart, bring your shoulders up to your ears as you inhale.
- Hold the pose for 10 seconds.
- Exhale and bring shoulders down slowly.
- Repeat the shrugging movement several times.

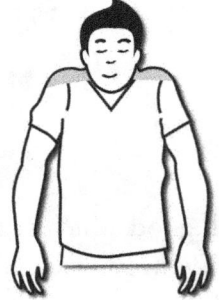

Neck Twist and Roll

- In a standing position, feet shoulder-width apart, inhale as you turn your head to the left as far as comfortable and hold for a few seconds.
- Exhale and return to face forward.
- Repeat on the right side.
- Repeat on both sides several times, always keeping the movement slow and controlled.
- Next, inhale and look up to the ceiling and exhale as you slowly make a half circle, clockwise with your nose until you're looking at the floor, then inhale as you complete the circle.
- Repeat anticlockwise.
- Alternate the motion several times.

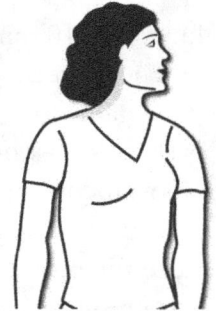

Ankle & Wrist Rolls

- Stand with your feet hip-width apart.
- Lift your right foot a few inches (use the wall for support if your balance is poor).
- Make a circle, as large as you can, with your toes in a clockwise motion several times, rotating the ankle joint.
- Repeat anticlockwise.
- Repeat on the other leg.

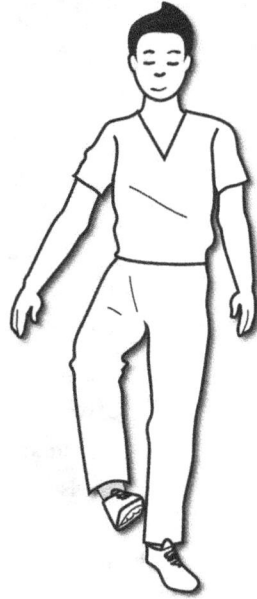

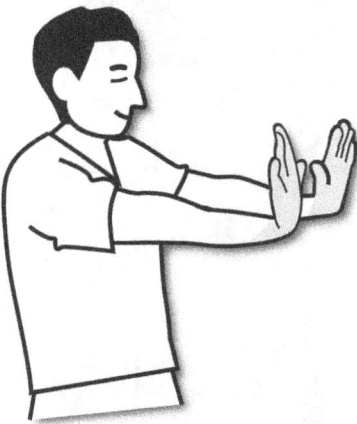

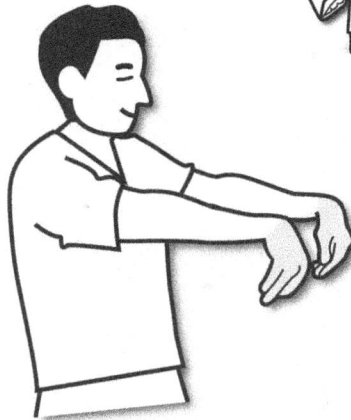

For wrist rolls, lift your arms forward to shoulder height and roll both wrists simultaneously for one minute and then change direction for another minute (listen to that clicking!).

Upward Salute

A great stretch for the intercostal and upper back muscles.

- Stand with your feet together, big toes touching.
- Arms are by your side, palms facing forwards.
- Imagine a thread is attached to the top of your head and gently pulling you up, so your spine is straight.
- Take a deep breath in as you arc your arms outwards from your body, lifting your hands above your head (palms should face each other).
- Look upwards through the gap between your hands (your spine should arc backwards gently).
- Don't scrunch up your shoulders; try to keep them relaxed.
- Keep looking up, breathing continuous deep, slow breaths.
- When you feel sufficiently stretched, lower your head to look forwards, then lower your arms.
- Stand for a few moments with your arms by your side as you began.

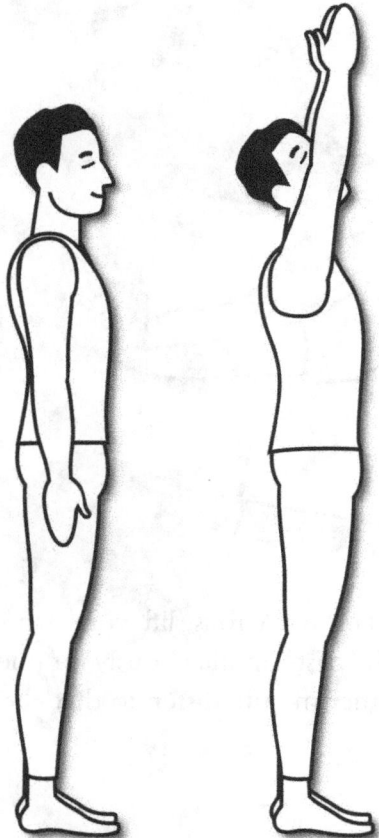

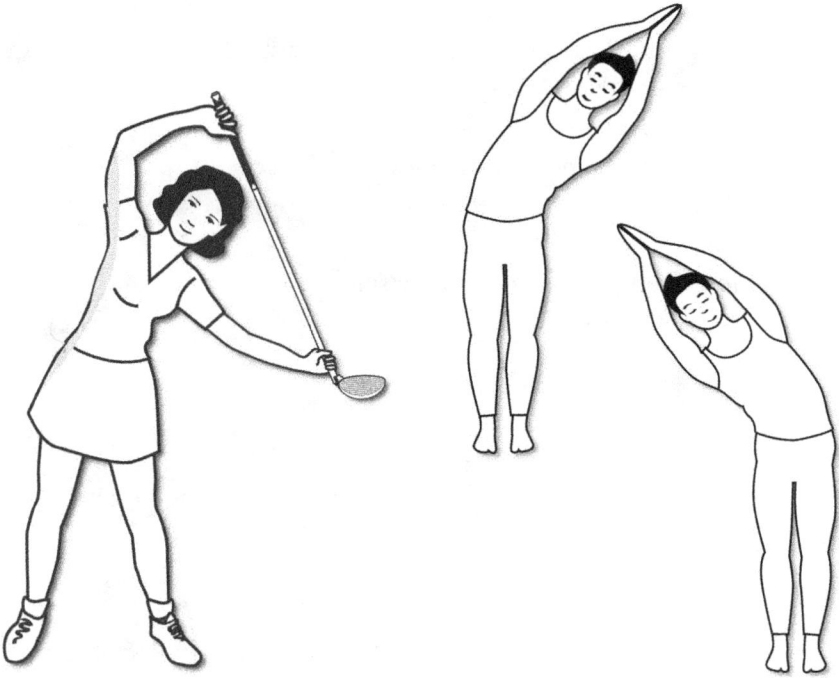

Side Stretch

A great stretch for the intercostal muscles.
- Do an upward salute but look forwards instead of upwards.
- When your arms are above your head, lean as far as you can to one side without changing the equal weight distribution in your feet.
- Keep your biceps close to your ears.
- Hold the pose for 30 seconds (don't forget to breathe!).
- Return to center for a moment or two and repeat the pose leaning the other way.
- Repeat both sides.

Hang Loose

- For a gentle lower back and hamstring stretch, stand with your feet hip-width apart.
- Bend forward from the waist.
- Let your head and arms hang down loosely.
- Hold the pose for 30 seconds (don't forget to keep breathing deeply and slowly).
- One vertebra at a time, slowly stand up straight.

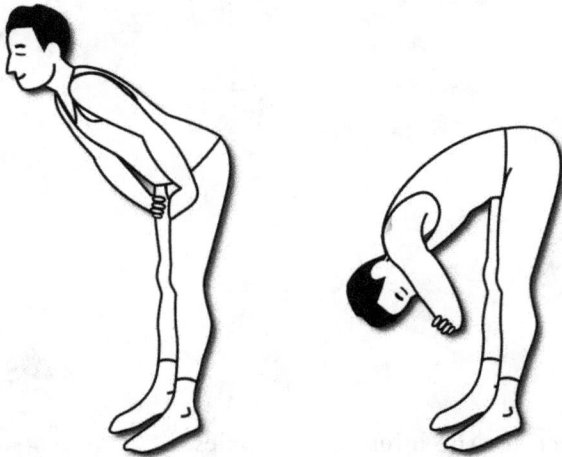

Recumbent & Railroad Stretches

These exercises improve posture and blood circulation, ease tension in the muscles, and strengthen the lungs.

- Lying on the floor with your arms by your sides, flex the ankles as if standing on the floor.
- Inhale as you slowly raise your arms to a perpendicular position, hold for several seconds, breathing deeply (recumbent stretch).

- Inhale again as you move your arms back another 90 degrees, palms facing each other, so that you are as flat on the floor as possible (railroad stretch).
- Exhale as you return your arms to the perpendicular position, hold for a few seconds, and on another exhale, lower your arms to the floor.
- Repeat the sequence, aiming to get your hands a little closer to the floor in the railroad stretch.

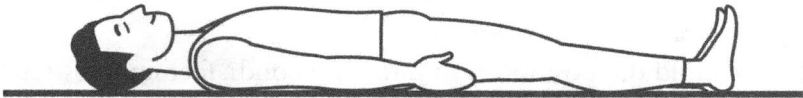

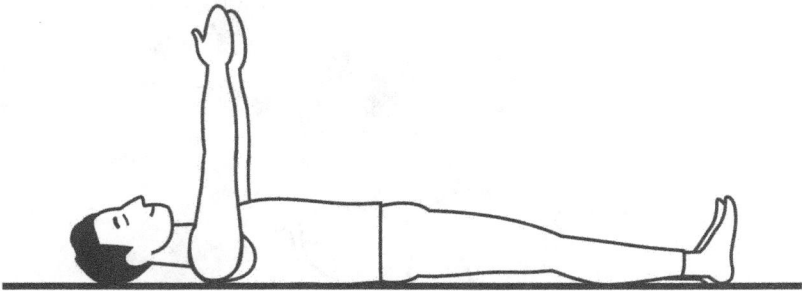

Butterfly Pose

This posture stretches the muscles in your inner thighs and lower back. The posture also improves the flexibility in the hips and spine; it also improves your digestion.

- Sit with the soles of your feet together and hold them with your hands.
- Allow your knees to relax towards the floor (don't force them) and inhale deeply.
- As you exhale, lower your head towards your feet, keeping your back as straight as possible.
- Draw in your abdomen.
- Hold the position for up to 15 seconds, feeling the stretch in your lower back.
- Inhale as you lift your head to sit up straight.
- Take a few breaths in the upright position, before repeating the back bend five or six times.

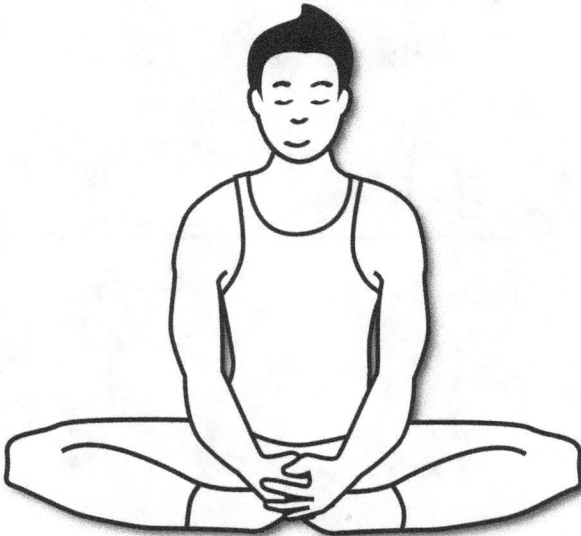

Chapter 4
STRENGTH & FLEXIBILITY

"You'll never grow old if you have a flexible spine."
—Yogi Bhajan.

Has anyone ever told you to loosen up? Well, it's good advice according to Yogi Bhajan, who tells us in his book *Kundalini Yoga* that we need both a flexible spine and a flexible attitude. He says that when the spine is rigid, the body's energy can't flow freely. And the key to flexibility is the spine, which is the control center for the 72,000 nerves in the body, which derive energy from the vertebrae.

When you wake in the morning, you may experience pain in your legs, hips, knees, and back. This discomfort may be because you are not exercising the right muscles, and it is perhaps a result of spending too much time sitting in cars or at desks with inadequate back support. This causes our muscles and joints to become stiff and our tendons to tighten.

Many weekend golfers tend to experience pain and play poorly as a result. They think that is because their swing mechanics are poor; however, the truth might just be that the pain is a result of inflexibility and weakness in the upper body. Blasting a golf ball between 60 and 90 times during a game will cause muscle fatigue and soreness, especially if you're not in good physical condition. Therefore, playing poorly is not necessarily something that requires a swing coach to fix. In many cases, players are much better off consulting a physical fitness coach and working on their strength, flexibility, and mobility to improve their golf swing. Of course, if you're developing your fitness but the pain continues, I suggest you stop all activity and consult a medical doctor.

Having warmed up with stretches, you're ready to take on some more physically demanding exercises. These will build your arm and shoulder muscles as well as your core strength. Building muscles in your core will protect you from injuries associated with a poor swing.

Ball Games

The weight ball is a useful tool for conditioning the shoulders, legs, core, glutes, and upper body. Do the following exercises daily and soon your waistband will be looser! But if you find them very painful, adapt them to suit your ability and build up from your own baseline.

1. Lifts

All of these exercises can be adapted to a prone position (lying on your back) and lifting the ball from your chest either toward the ceiling or the wall behind you.

Using a lightweight ball of between 5 and 8 pounds, start in a standing position and hold the ball in the middle of your chest. Slowly lift the ball above your head, fully extending your arms. Do this movement at least 20 times per set and do 3 to 5 sets. Hold your stomach muscles tight as you do this exercise to build your core strength. Inhale to lift, exhale to return to the starting position. Make sure you take the 20-count rest between sets.

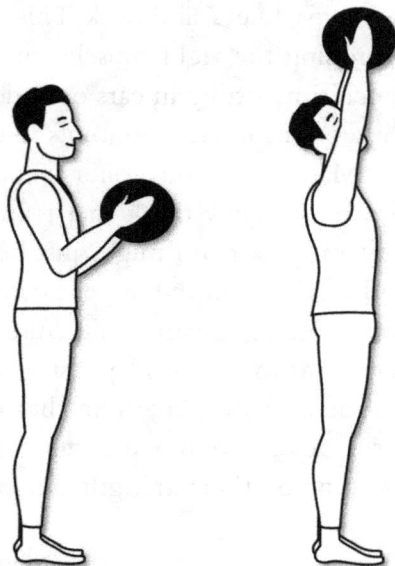

Next, lift the ball above your head and hold it there for a count of 50. Bring the ball back to your chest and relax for a count of 20. Repeat this movement at least 3 times. Don't forget to hold the stomach muscles tight during the lifts. Inhale to lift and exhale to return to the starting position.

As you get stronger, lift the ball above your head and hold it for as long as possible (keeping the stomach muscles tight). When you cannot keep it aloft any longer, lower the ball to the chest and count to 20 before lifting again. Do this at least 3 times. Inhale to lift, breathing normally, and exhale to return to the starting position.

If you are in a prone sitting position, as you lift the ball up to the ceiling or over your head, raise your feet about 6 to 8 inches from the floor, keeping your legs straight. Hold this position for as long as you have the ball in the air. Be sure that you inhale as you lift and exhale as you return to the start position.

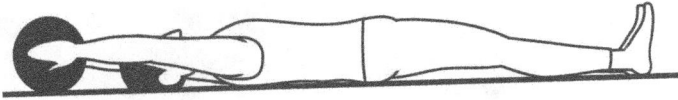

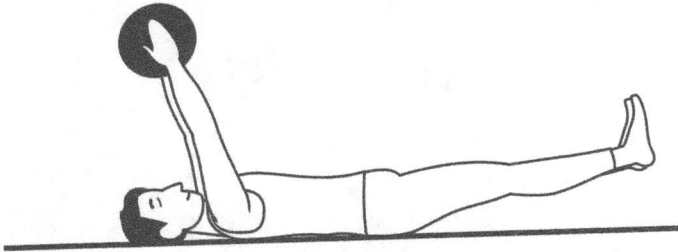

2. Squats

Using an 8-pound ball, stand with your back to a wall and hold out the ball. Lower yourself to a sitting position using the wall for support. Hold this position for a count of 20 (as you get stronger, this count will increase), while bringing the ball into your chest and out again, 10 times per set. Do at least 3 sets to start.

Next, bring the ball to your chest and lift it above your head, hold the position for a count of 30 and return to the starting position. Repeat this movement between 3 and 5 times. As you become stronger, you can hold the position for as long as you like. Remember to inhale for the lift and breathe normally until you return to the starting position and then exhale. Keep your core muscles tight during these exercises.

Now for some yoga. The following yoga poses will develop stronger and suppler wrist, knee, and elbow joints, as well as greater flexibility in your spine.

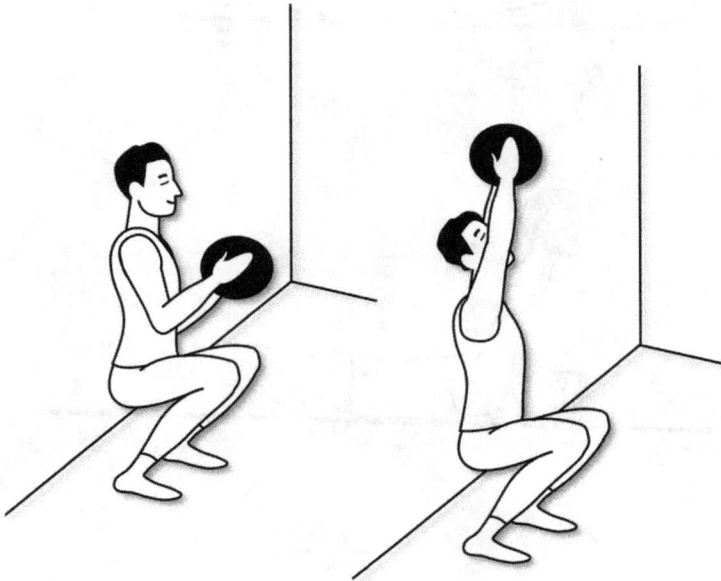

Cat-Cow

This is a gentle sequence that keeps the spine supple; it is also a gentle weight-bearing exercise for your arms and shoulders. You should keep a blanket nearby in case you need some extra padding to protect your knees.

- Start on your hands and knees.
- Your knees should be directly under your hips and your hands directly under your shoulders.
- Inhale as you lower your abdomen towards the mat and lift your tailbone.
- Look upwards, creating a nice downwards arc with your spine.
- Exhale as you round your back and tuck your head and tailbone in.
- Hold for a few seconds, pulling your navel towards your spine.
- Repeat several times.

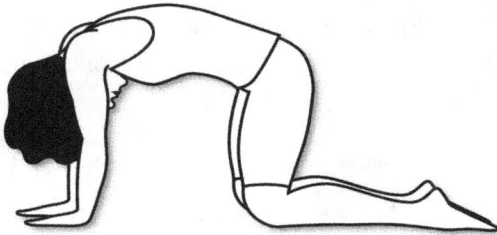

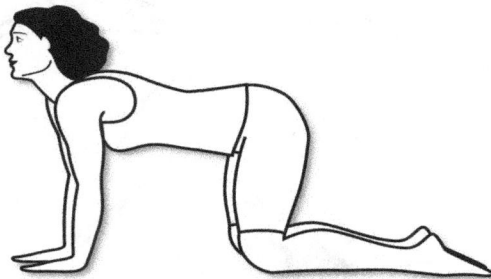

Downward Dog

Downward Dog is a fundamental yoga pose that you will probably do several times during a yoga class. This is a good stretch for the hamstrings and Achilles tendons, and it is a more intense weight-bearing exercise, making for stronger hands, wrists, arms, and shoulders.

- Start on your hands and knees, aligned as in Cat-Cow.
- Spread your fingers so that your weight is evenly distributed in your hands.
- On the inhale, raise your tailbone.
- Straighten your legs and lower your heels to the floor as much as you can.
- Your back should be as straight as possible.
- Relax your neck.
- Bend and flex the knees alternately to gently stretch the backs of your legs.
- Don't forget to keep breathing deeply.
- Hold the pose for as long as possible.
- Rest in Child's Pose (see the chapter on relaxation) between poses.
- Repeat five or six times.

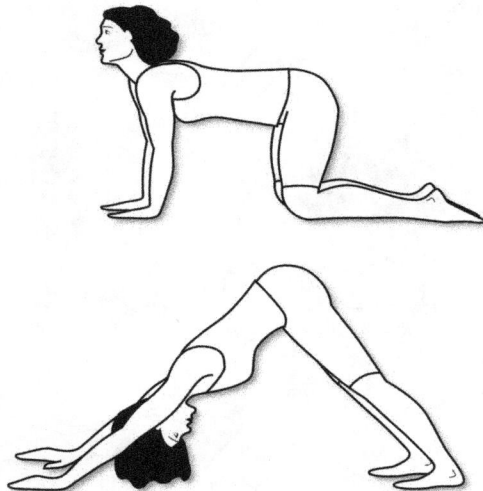

Plank Pose

This is one of the transition poses and is featured mainly the Sun Salutation sequence. It strengthens the arms, shoulders, wrists, legs, ankles, back, and core. If you can't hold this posture, you can rest on your forearms instead of your hands.

- Start in Downward Dog.
- Lower your tailbone as you step both feet back so that the plane of your body from your head to your heels is as straight as possible.
- Keep your hands below your shoulders.
- Pull your navel towards your spine.
- Keep breathing deeply and evenly as you hold the pose for 30 seconds.
- Drop your knees to the floor and rest in Child's Pose.

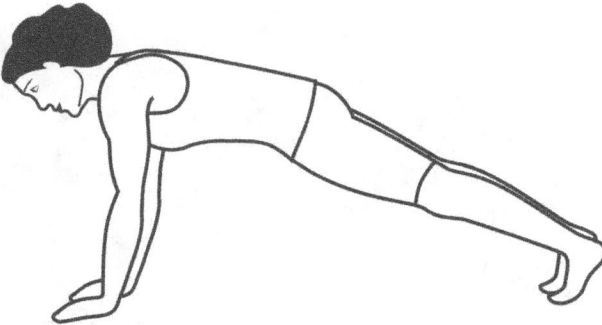

High Lunge

This pose strengthens the legs and stretches the groin. It is also good for digestion and sciatica.

- From a standing pose, step one foot back as far as you can.
- Bend the front knee to a right angle, moving your hands to the floor either side of your front leg (use blocks if necessary).
- All your weight should be in your feet (your hands should be used only for balance).
- Keep the back leg as straight as possible (as in Plank, the line from your head to your heel should be straight).
- Pull in your navel toward your spine and hold the pose for 30 seconds.
- On the inhale, bring your back foot to meet your front one, and on the exhale move your other foot back to repeat the pose on the other side (rest between left and right pose if necessary).

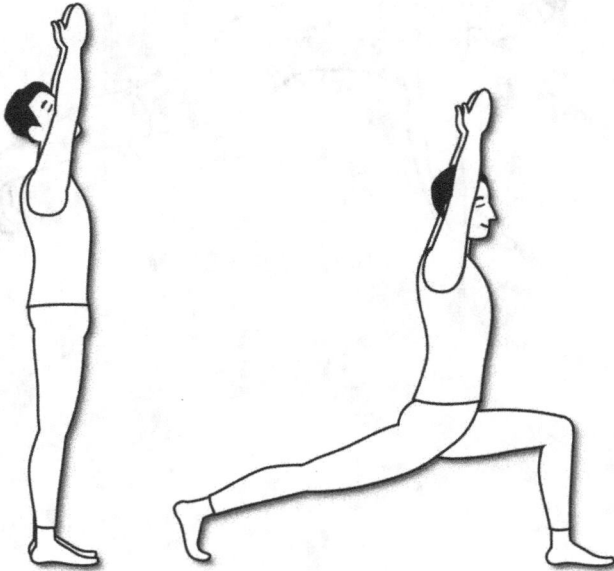

Staff Pose

This looks like a simple pose, but it works your back muscles hard and strengthens your core.

- Sit on the mat with your legs outstretched.
- Pull your toes back towards you.
- Keep your legs and spine as straight as possible, creating a right angle between your torso and thighs.
- Place your hands on the mat beside your hips.
- Pull your navel towards your spine.
- Imagine a thread is pulling at the top of your head as you breathe deeply and evenly, holding the pose for a minute.

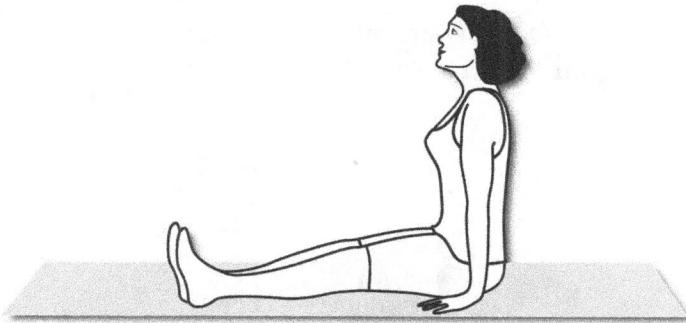

Seated Twist

This pose is a good for your spine's flexibility.

- Sitting in Staff Pose, lift your right knee, keeping your left leg straight.
- Cross your bent leg over your straight leg so that your foot is against your left outer knee.
- Hook your left arm over your bent knee, your elbow pressing against the bent leg to keep it in position.
- On the inhale, twist your torso as far as you can, looking over your right shoulder.
- Breathe deeply and evenly.
- Pull in your stomach to twist further and hold the pose for 30 seconds.
- Return to face forward and release your arm and knee.
- Repeat on the other side.

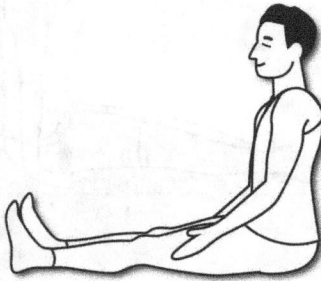

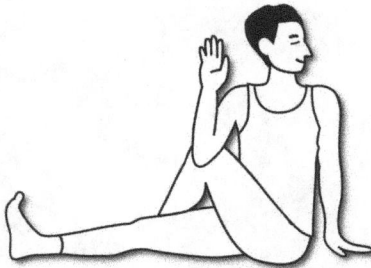

Recumbent Staff Pose

This exercise is most beneficial when it comes after the Recumbent Stretch. It is an intense pose that is a great way to strengthen your core and your back muscles. It also good for hip flexibility.

- Lie on the floor with feet together and hands at your sides.
- Inhale as you slowly raise your legs so that they are perpendicular to the floor (a Recumbent Staff Pose).
- Hold the pose for 10 to 60 seconds (continue deep, even breathing).
- Exhale while you are lowering your legs to the floor.
- Repeat as many times as is comfortable.

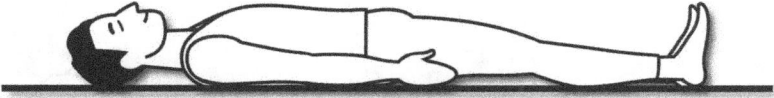

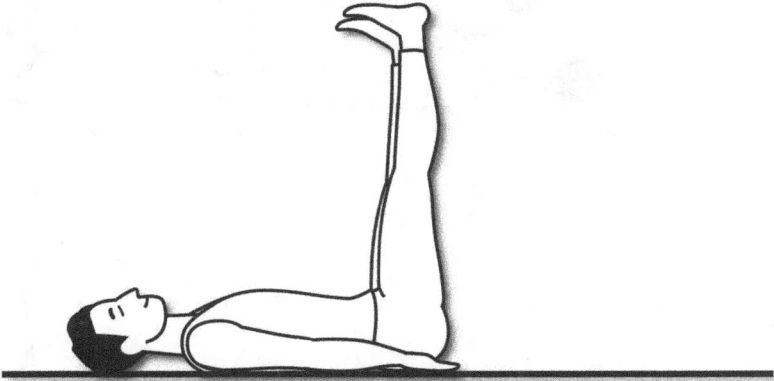

Bridge Pose

This pose strengthens the leg and gluteal muscles and increases the flexibility of the spine. It also stretches and relieves tension of the upper back and neck.

- Lie on your back with your knees bent and your feet hip–width apart (try touching your heels with your fingertips).
- Inhale, tighten your buttocks and slowly lift your pelvis, lower, and middle back so that it forms a straight line to your kneecaps.
- Press your upper back and shoulders firmly into the floor.
- Hold this position for at least 60 seconds.
- Exhale and lower yourself slowly, one vertebra at a time.
- Relax and repeat this pose several times.

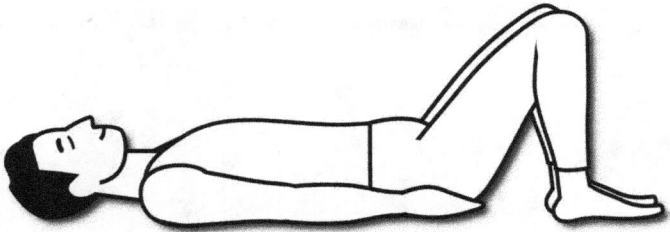

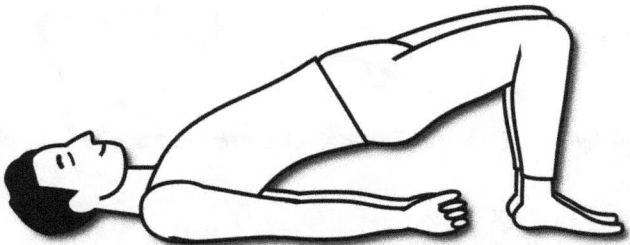

Chair Pose

Strengthens and stretches the ankles, spine, thighs, and arms. It also stretches the chest and shoulders. The longer you practice, the lower you will be able to get in the pose. Do not do this pose if you have knee problems, and if it hurts, STOP!

- Start from standing position, feet a few inches apart.
- Keeping your hands at your sides, bend your knees as far as is comfortable.
- As you start to squat, inhale and bring your hands together.
- Raise your hands above your head.
- Hold this position for as long as you can, at least to a count of 50.

To take this pose one step further, get into the Chair Pose position and then twist so that your left elbow is resting on your right knee.

- Keep breathing and hold the pose for several seconds.
- On an exhale, twist the other way so that the right elbow is touching the left knee.
- Hold the pose, release, and repeat.

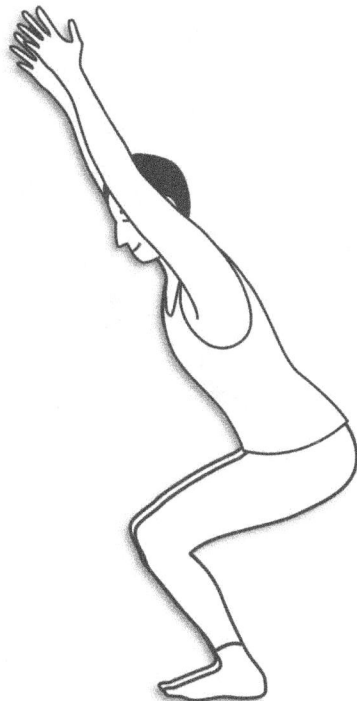

Chapter 5

BALANCE & POSTURE

It is important to pay attention to each step in the yoga process to achieve the balance between the mind and the body. The reason that it's pleasurable to listen to a great love song, or read a love poem, is that there is a sense of rhythm and harmony. This is the same with yoga. It is important to strive for a balance between the physical and psychological. The poses in this section develop your physical balance, and the chapter on relaxation and meditation works to develop the balance within your mind.

Physical balance is essential to your golf game because it affects your posture. In 2003, I attended a seminar delivered by Dr. Jeffrey H. Blanchard, which had a huge impact on my game, raising my handicap from a 16 to a 3. Blanchard says: "Posture over the golf ball plays an enormous role in influencing swing traits such as body coil to generate power and accurate maintenance of the golf club along the circular and incline plane during the golf swing."

The balancing poses described below are also great for improving your posture because they all require straight spines. Yoga poses should be performed without shoes and socks, and this is especially important in the balancing poses because it will enable you to feel the correctness of the posture through your feet.

Mountain Pose

This forms the foundation of many standing poses. This posture straightens the spine, improves posture, tones the buttocks, and strengthens the ankles and legs. It is also helpful in achieving a balance of the body and mind. Most people are unaware that they are not standing in a balanced position and that this affects the alignment of the entire body. By practicing this posture, you will develop your sense of steadiness, firmness, and strength in your entire body.

- Stand with your big toes touching.
- Extend both arms straight down, with palms inward, fingers together and pointing toward the floor.
- Tuck in your tailbone and tighten your quadriceps and gluteal muscles and lift the kneecaps.
- Your spine and head should be in a straight line and your shoulders slightly back to broaden the chest.
- Tighten the muscles in your neck slightly without straining.
- Hold this position for at least 30 seconds.
- Breathe normally during this exercise.

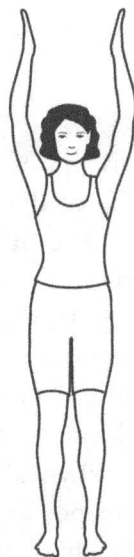

As a variation, stand against a wall (to improve alignment):

- Starting with your palms facing outward, inhale as you raise your arms above your head.
- Try touching the wall above you with your palms, with your arms as straight as possible.
- You should feel the stretch through your wrists, fingers, and both sides of your body.
- Hold this for a count of 30, pulling in your lower abdomen.
- Exhale and relax your arms back down to your side.
- Repeat this posture several times and feel the spine relax.

Squat Pose

Squatting is, in fact, the most natural position for our bodies. There are many cultures throughout the world in which people spend a lot of time squatting as opposed to sitting in chairs, but it requires balance. In addition to developing balance, a squat can build strength in the muscles and joints in our knees, back, legs, ankles, hips, and our core.

- Test your squatting ability first by standing with your feet together.
- Raise your arms above your head.
- Keeping your back and arms straight and your heels on the floor, bend your knees and lower your sitting bones.
- If you can sit on your heels, you're in great shape, but if you can only lower yourself a little, you can develop your ability by using a wall.
- Stand against a smooth wall with your arms lifted above your head.
- Keeping your heels together and close to the wall, slowly slide your bottom downwards until you are in a sitting position.
- Hold the position for 30 seconds, breathing deeply and evenly.
- Inhale and then slide back up the wall as you exhale.
- Repeat at least 3 times, each time holding for 30 seconds.
- Each time you attempt the pose, try to get closer to your heels, and as you get stronger, try to do it without the wall.

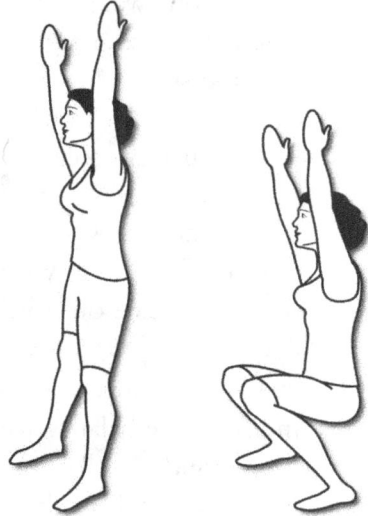

Tree Pose

In addition to improving your balance, Tree Pose will strengthen your legs and stretch your inner thighs. If your balance is terrible, you can begin by doing the pose with your back to the wall.

- Stand with your feet slightly apart and feel grounded.
- Adjust your weight gradually to your right foot and slowly lift your left.
- Rest your right sole against your ankle or calf muscle (never rest your foot on your knee) with your bent knee out to the side.
- Press your palms together and hold the balance for a few seconds.
- When you feel steady enough, lift your arms above your head.
- For a more advanced pose, take hold of your foot and lift it above the knee joint of the standing leg and press it against your upper thigh.
- Press your palms together, then lift your arms above your head, and hold the balance (if your foot slips, you can use a belt to keep it in place).

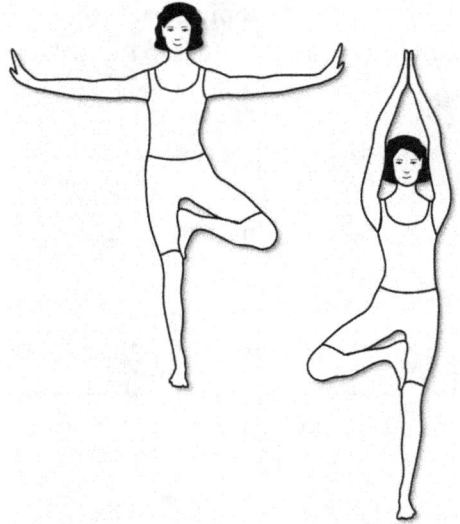

Extended Triangle Pose

This is principally a stretching pose, but balance also plays a huge part.

- Stand with your feet together and move your right foot back about 3.5 to 4 feet.
- Raise your arms out to the sides, level with your shoulders, palms down.
- Turn your front foot inward slightly and turn your back foot out 90 degrees.
- Shift your feet to ensure that both heels are in alignment.
- Imagine you're reaching for something with your right hand and, on an exhale, bend forward from the hip (not the waist).
- Lower your right hand to the floor (or a block).
- Your left arm should be straight up so that there is a line from the right hand on the floor to the left hand in the air.
- Your torso should be in line with your forward leg (you shouldn't be leaning forward).
- If it's not a strain on your neck, look up at your hand.
- Repeat on your left side.

If you feel as if you're falling backwards in this pose, you can do it against a wall until your balance improves.

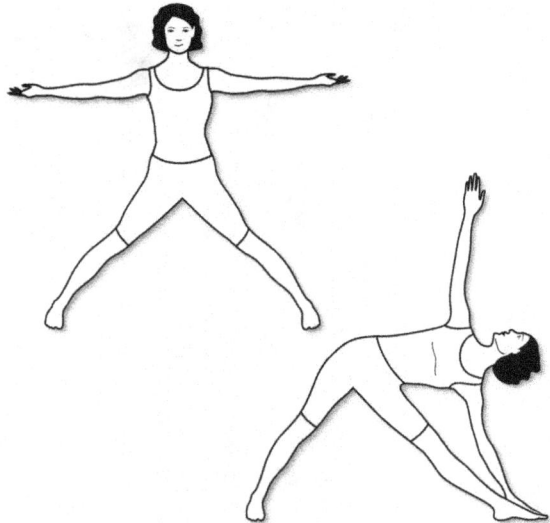

Half Moon Pose

This is one step on from the previous pose. In addition to helping your balance, it also builds strength in your legs and arms, and improves hip flexibility.

- Perform the Extended Triangle Pose but put your right hand on your right hip.
- Bend the front knee slightly and touch the floor (or block) with your left hand.
- Straighten the bent knee and lift your back leg out straight behind you.
- Raise your right arm so it forms a line with your left arm.
- Look at your right hand, if it's not a strain on the neck.
- Hold the pose for 30 seconds.
- Repeat on the other side.

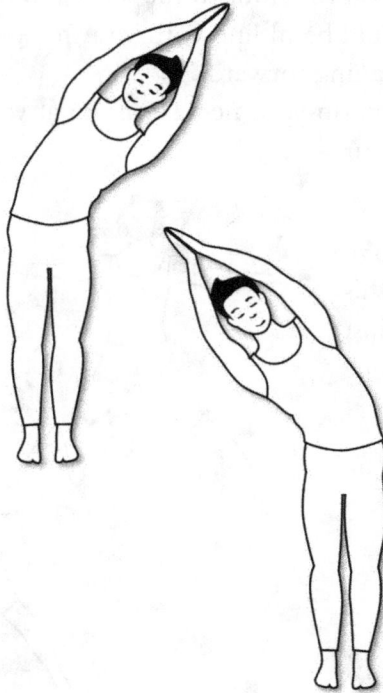

Archer Pose

This pose improves flexibility and strengthens the feet, knees, legs and ankles. It also opens the hip joints and elongates the spine. It is also great for endurance and stamina.

- Stand facing forward.
- Step the right leg back as far as is comfortable (your back foot should be at a 45-degree angle to help with stability).
- Keeping your spine totally straight, bend the knee of the front leg so that your knee is over your ankle (no further) and your thigh is parallel to the floor. The deeper you bend your knee the better.
- Making a fist with your left hand, raise your left arm parallel to the floor.
- Fold your right arm and lift from the shoulder so the elbow is pointing directly behind you (as if pulling on a bowstring); feel the stretch as you pull back the string of the bow.
- Your eyes should be looking straight ahead.
- Hold this pose for 1 to 2 minutes while deep breathing.
- Repeat the pose on the other side of your body.

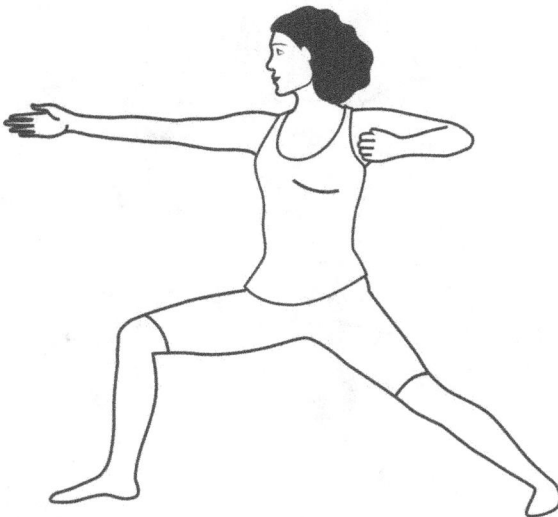

Garland Pose

This is another type of squat pose that requires balance. It is also a good stretch for the back and the groin.

- Stand with your feet together and squat on your heels (if your heels are off the floor, put a folded blanket under them for support.
- Maintain your balance while opening the knees wide, moving your feet to 45-degree angle.
- Press your palms together and keep your knees from coming together with your elbows.
- For extra balancing practice, extend your arms out to the side and hold for 30 seconds.

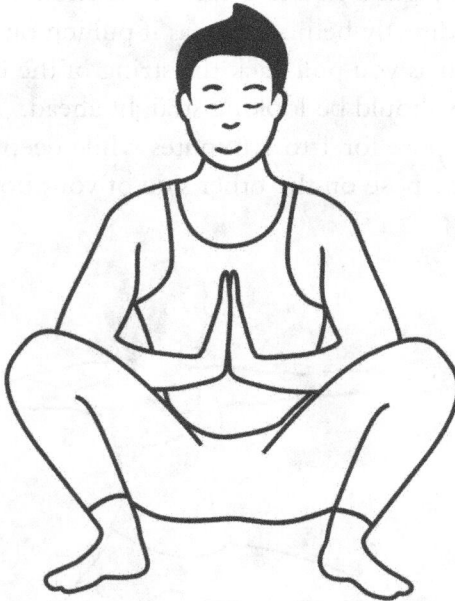

Chapter 6

RELAXATION & MEDITATION

"I've quit worrying about poor shots. I just tell myself, 'Relax, Bozo. If you can't have fun, you shouldn't be out here.'"
—Patty Sheehan, American pro golfer

I truly enjoy golf and have made many new friends by playing the game over the years. There were times it was great for doing business and staying in shape, and playing it felt good. However, there were other times when, due to stress involving personal relationships and work, I was not a happy person, and I was overwhelmed. What attracted me to yoga initially was the fact it was a positive way of dealing with all the strife and anger in my life. Yoga helped me personally, but it also helped my golf game.

When I played poorly sometimes, I would get frustrated and think I should just stop playing because it was no fun. But one bad hole does not a bad game make. One time, I was about to quit, when on the very next hole, I eagled a 420-yard, par-4 hole, hitting a 190-yard shot onto the green with a 7 iron. Needless to say, those kinds of shots can bring the sense of fun back! But not every shot goes well, and not every game is a success, so finding ways to take the rough with the smooth is essential.

Over the years, I have become aware that there is a spiritual component to the practice of yoga. When the body and mind work together properly, there are vibrations that have a positive impact on one's life. By practicing the relaxation and meditation aspects of yoga, you will quiet your doubting, analytical mind and learn to play golf for the sheer pleasure of doing so. Yoga attunes your sense to the peace and beauty of the course and the wonder of the present moment. When you are able to put away thoughts of failure, disappointment, and anxiety, you will then be able to fully enjoy playing—not in order to win or outdo your fellow players, but rather for the simple enjoyment and relaxation of the game.

In order to fully appreciate the game of golf, understand it with your head, believe it with your heart, and know it with you soul. Yoga is a path to attaining these three states of being.

US golfer Mark McCumber said, "It takes so long to accept that you can't always replicate your swing. The only thing you can control is your attitude toward the next shot." Yoga can give you an attitude adjustment that brings you into a peaceful state of mind, no matter what happened during your last shot or is about to happen on the next.

Relaxation

It is important to end your yoga practice with some relaxation poses, but it is also important that you stop and relax between poses during the yoga routine itself. Relax in a comfortable position with your eyes closed. Take a few deep breaths, and try not to think about anything for a few moments. Bring yourself back to the present moment. "Time out" will help calm you, reduce your heart rate, and allow you rest for a few moments before you begin again.

Poses

Relaxation poses—sometimes called restorative poses—are the most passive of the yoga positions. They often appear at the end of the class when participants are cooling down and meditating. One of the biggest challenges is stopping yourself from falling asleep. Don't be that person in the yoga class who snores throughout the relaxation part of the class!

Hero's Pose

I start and complete my yoga practice daily with this pose. It not only gives a nice stretch to the ankles, thighs and knees, it also helps relieve stress and relax the mind.

- In a kneeling position, sit on your heels with your knees together
- Place your hands on your thighs, fingers apart and relaxed
- Keep the back straight
- Breathe deeply
- Keep your eyes half closed, and try to clear your mind of all thoughts.

This is also a good pose in which to practice Breath of Fire (see the Breathing section below), which is powerful method for building a strong nervous system.

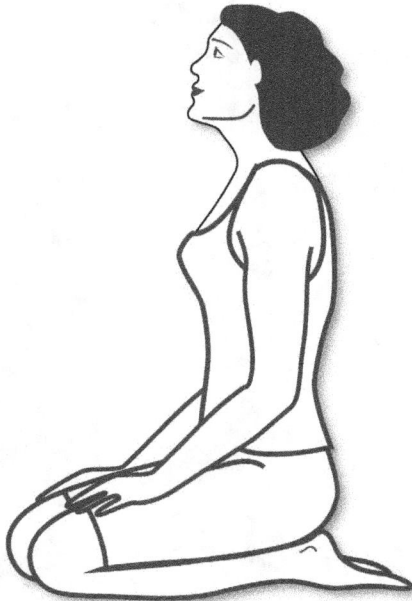

Forward Bend

Relieves physical and mental stress by slowing down the heart rate. It is also good for your organs, including the kidneys, spleen, and liver. The pose improves your balance while also relieving abdominal or back pain, and strengthening the legs, thighs, and ankles.

- Start in Mountain Pose.
- Inhale and lift your arms straight above your head with your hands forward.
- Lift your kneecaps.
- Exhale and bend at the waist without bending the knees.
- Bend as far forward as possible without pain (if you are able to touch your palms to the floor, you are in very good shape! Most of us require lots of practice to be able to touch the floor).
- Hold this posture for at least 20 seconds.
- Inhale and return to Mountain Pose.
- Breathe normally, relax, and repeat this posture several times, each time attempting to stretch further towards the floor.

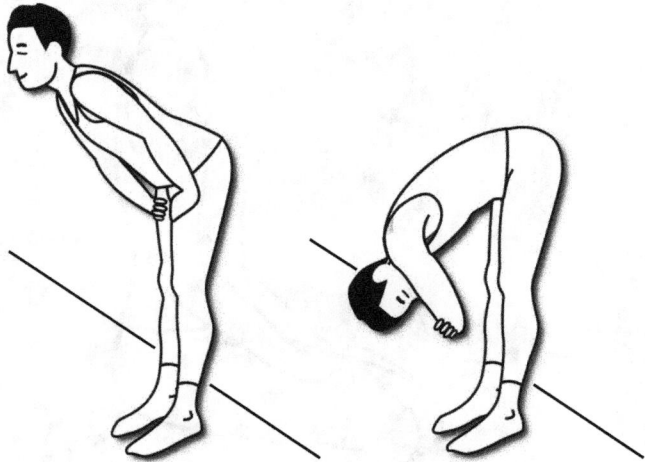

Child's Pose

This is a great pose when you need a rest during strenuous poses or some relaxation. Although it is a restorative pose, it still requires the active use of the arms. It is good for the knee and hip joints.

- In a kneeling position, widen your knees to the edges of your mat but keep your feet together.
- Lean forward and stretch out your arms as far as you can in front of you.
- Press your hands lightly into the mat.
- Rest your forehead on the floor.
- Hold the pose, keeping your back as straight as possible and breathing deeply and evenly.

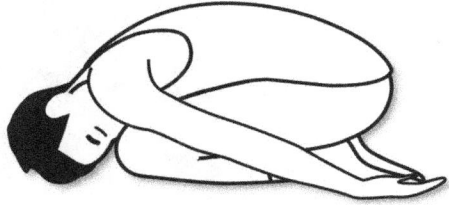

Legs Up the Wall

More advanced students of yoga might do inversions, which include head, shoulder, and hand stands. The Legs Up the Wall pose is a kind of inversion that beginners can do as an alternative to fully inverted poses, and it's much more relaxing.

- Sit with one hip pressed against the wall.
- Lower yourself onto your side, ensuring that your bottom stays in contact with the wall.
- Roll onto your back so that your legs are vertical, your heels are against the wall, and your toes are pointing into the room.
- Shuffle your bottom as close to the wall as possible.
- If you have tight hamstrings, put a folded blanket or bolster under you bottom.
- Let your arms relax, palms facing upward, fingers relaxed.

- Close your eyes and hold the pose for as long as you like.
- To come out of the pose, bend your knees towards your chest, roll to one side, and slowly sit upright.

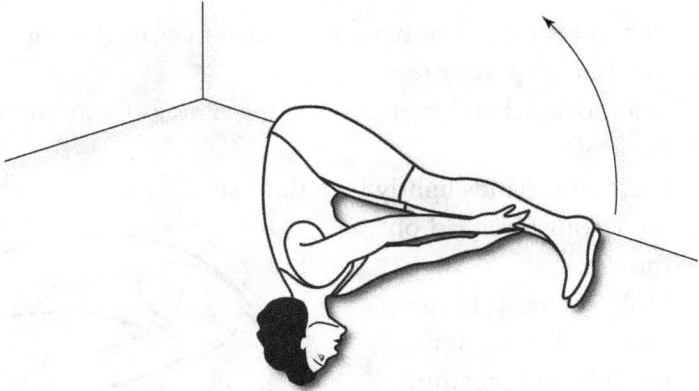

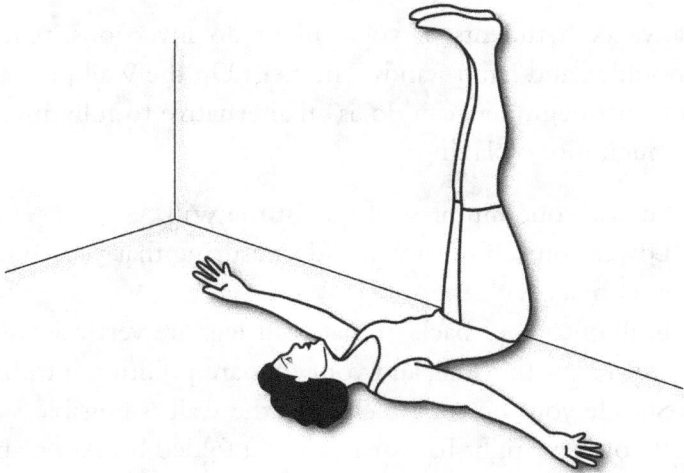

Extended Puppy Pose

This pose relaxes the brain and reduces stress to the nervous system, which assists in calming the mind and rejuvenating the entire body. In addition, it lengthens the spine and stretches the shoulders and arms. This is a great pose to do after several repetitions of Downward Dog.

- Begin on your hands and knees (hands should be shoulder-width apart and your knees under your hips).
- Inhale and walk your hands away from your body, bringing your head down to the floor.
- Let your abdomen support your lower back as you allow the neck muscles to relax.
- Hold this movement for as longs as it feels good.
- Breathe softly and just relax.

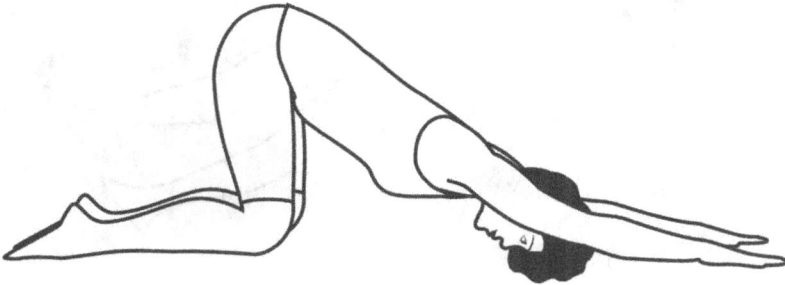

Corpse Pose

This morbidly named posture may seem simple, but it requires something we're not used to: stillness. The pose helps you relieve tension and clear your mind.

- Simply lie on your back.
- Legs apart, feet flopped out to the side.
- Arms away from your body, palms up, fingers relaxed.
- Close your eyes and focus on every part of your body from head to toe, making sure you relax every muscle and joint.
- Don't forget to relax your facial, neck, and stomach muscles (we unconsciously keep these tight).

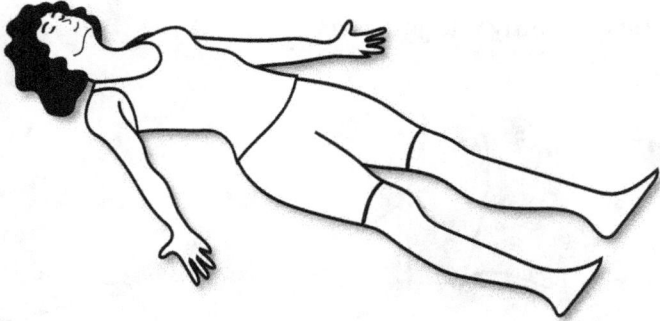

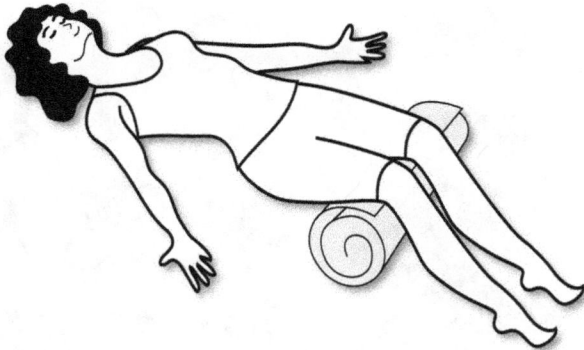

Breathing

Don't take this part of your life for granted. Your breath is your best friend. It comes with you at birth and stays with you all of your life.

Your boyfriends, girlfriends husbands, wives, and best friends can come and go. But, your breath stay with you no matter what happens in your life.

When one dies, they inhale, hoping that they might get one more breath. Learn how to properly use your breath, then you and your breath, will be together for a lifetime, no matter what.

If you ask someone what the most important aspect of a great sporting performance is, few would say "breathing." This is because most of us don't spend much time thinking about the act of breathing—after all, it comes so naturally. But athletes—from runners to swimmers to football players—know that when they learn to breathe properly, their performance is enhanced.

Learning yoga is a great way for golfers to improve their breathing. Better breathing will help their swing and lower their anxiety or frustration.

The word hatha means "sun" *(ha)* and "moon" *(tha)*, and the breath work involved in yoga also reflects this duality: An inhalation through the right nostril is called the "sun breath" and through the left, "moon breath." The hatha yogi learns to regulate the breath and bring harmony from the sun and the moon into his or her life.

In general, breathing exercises aid relaxation, self-healing, and focus. Effective breathing strengthens muscles and improves movement in the joints, allowing them to stretch further.

Proper breathing is as important to the golfer as balance or strength. In fact, proper breathing helps when the golfer is at the tee because it helps him or her relax and focus. You can control your mind by controlling your breathing. The mind follows the breath and the body follows the mind. Master your breath and your mind, and you will master your body. In his book *The Flow of Eternal Power,* Yogi Bhajan states: "The mind becomes a monster when it becomes your master. The mind is an angel when it is your servant."

In my very first Kundalini class, we spent an hour learning to breathe. I remember thinking that was a bit much, given that I'd been breathing my whole life! But that hour opened my eyes to the importance of breathing *properly*. With each breath, I felt myself relax—so much so that I wanted to sleep. But you must remain awake to concentrate on the inhale and exhale. In yoga, the name for the inhale is *prana* and the name for exhale is *apana*.

Yoga incorporates three types of breathing:

- Belly breathing (diaphragmatic): The diaphragm contracts and the abdomen expands (good for the abdomen).
- Intercostal breathing (athletic respiration): The rib cage moves up and the chest expands. It is a shallow breathing that utilizes the middle part of the lungs.
- Clavicular breathing: A shallow breathing that draws air into the lungs using the intercostal muscles rather than the diaphragm.

In order to get more in touch with your breath and feel what proper breathing is, follow this simple exercise:

- Lie on your back.
- Place your hands lightly at the base of your rib cage and exhale as much air from your lungs as possible.
- Then inhale as deeply as possible. Notice how your hands rise and fall with each breath.
- With each inhale, fill your abdomen, then let the breath fill your lungs. When you exhale, allow the breath to escape from the lungs first and then deflate your abdomen, pulling in your belly, letting all the air out.
- Feel each breath in your lower and upper chest.

Breath walks are a great way to get in shape and enjoy nature at the same time. During this exercise, be aware of the way you breathe more than the way you walk. Some types of breathing are outlined below.

1. **Slow & Easy Breathing**

   Inhale for a count of 10 seconds, hold your breath for 10 seconds, and exhale for 10 seconds.

   This relaxed breathing eases you into your conditioning. On the golf course, use this technique of counting breaths and steps to keep your mind off the last hole and on the present moment.

2. **Fire Breathing**

   This exercise helps you build stamina. Walk as fast as you can for as far as you can. Inhale and exhale with each step you take. It's okay to start slowly and build up your breathing, your stamina, and your speed. By effectively using the fire walk, you will deliver more oxygen to your body, thereby improving lung function and stimulating blood circulation.

3. **Alternate Nostril Breathing**

   Because this exercise increases the amount of oxygen available to the body, use it before any strenuous activity, not just a game of golf.

   Using your thumb and little finger of your left hand (tucking in the other fingers), close your right nostril with the little finger and inhale through the open left nostril. Hold your breath, then release your right nostril and simultaneously close your left nostril with your thumb to let out the breath. When the full breath has been released, keep your thumb on your left nostril and inhale through the right, and hold your breath again. To exhale, move the little finger back to the right nostril, closing it for the out-breath. Repeat several times for 1 to 3 minutes.

   You can use this technique on the golf course as you walk between the holes, or to your ball, if you have a free hand. Because it requires some concentration, it will keep your mind focused on the present moment. Or you can use it before you begin the game: You'll be amazed by how much energy it gives you.

4. **Attitude Breathing**

There are times in our daily life that we become over stressed had by something or another and it appear that we may fall apart. When we are on the Golf Course and have a bad shot. That short could take over our entire being might even cost the entire game.

There is a breathing technique that I use to bring myself back into the present. I call the breathing technique.

Attitude Breathing:

1: Inhale deeply while counting 25 (25 Seconds)
2: Hold for 10 seconds
3: Exhale while counting to 25 (25 Seconds)
Repeat this process twice:

While doing so all you will be able to do is think about your breathing and by doing so you will release all the stress that the moment has created and then you will able to return to your next shot without thinking about the last shot. This a very good process for being mindful.

This breathing technique, can work as well in your daily life, by controlling what is going on around you, you remain mindful.

I have used this breathing process in the Boardroom as well as on the Golf Course!

Meditation

"May your life's stroll always be down the middle
With an execution of approaches tried and true
While watching the rolling putts drop magically
Under radiant skies of a majestic blue."
—Golfer's Prayer

The short prayer above was written by perhaps the most well-known caddie of all time, Aggie Cross, and it is not only a nice way to start this section but also every game! Of course, prayer is a form of meditation, and if you are of a religious nature, you will be well prepared to try the exercises below.

Energy is one of the most important elements of life, and it's essential to playing any sport. The best way to boost your energy is with proper food, well-developed breathing habits, peaceful sleep, and regular meditation.

Like yoga, meditation comes in many forms. Here are a few.

Transcendental Meditation®

Uses sound mantras (chanting). It was introduced by Maharishi Mahesh Yogi in the mid-1950s. It is practiced twice a day for about 15 minutes.

Heart Rhythm Meditation

Focuses on conscious breathing. It is a method that was first described in a 2008 book by Puran Bair called *Living from the Heart*.

Guided Visualization (or Guided Imagery)

Is a method that involves using the "mind's eye" to envision a place of natural beauty. It usually takes place in a relaxing atmosphere with music, scent, and soft light, and it is "guided" by a practitioner who prompts pleasant thoughts. This is a good type of meditation for golfers because it teaches them to visualize the ideal shot (the flight and destination of the ball).

Qigong

Is a physical method of meditation, involving slow, flowing movements and deep, rhythmic breathing. Qigong translates as "life energy cultivation." The practice originated in China.

Zazen

A seated meditation. It is a Zen Buddhist practice, usually performed in the Lotus Position (crossed legged). The meditation involves focusing on oneself and achieving harmony with one's surroundings.

Mindfulness Meditation (my personal favorite)

Also comes from the Buddhist tradition and is a sitting meditation, like zazen. Originally, it was a way to relieve suffering, which, thankfully, not many of us experience to extreme degrees anymore. But it is a useful way to overcome the small, everyday trials and tribulations of life (and golf). This is the kind of meditation that golfers can get the most benefit from. As thoughts arise, you acknowledge them nonjudgmentally before letting them pass. Ten to 15 minutes is usually sufficient, but some can meditate for up to an hour.

For me, mindfulness meditation helps me avoid daily stress professionally and personally. It is not easy to be mindful—it takes time and practice. I have been working on it for several years, and I now know that by "staying in the moment," great things happen.

Despite my determination, however, I have by no means fully mastered the art of mindfulness! Recently, I was invited to play golf with some friends at a course I had never played. It started out well, but, on a long par-5 hole, there was a lake to the right of the fairway. I tried to keep my mind off it as I hit a great drive . . . right into the water hazard. The only thing I was mindful of in that moment was how badly I played that hole, which totally threw me off my game! It took me several more holes to make an eagle and get back to staying in the moment. Remember that the more you practice, the better you will be able to control your mind and your life.

Yogi Bajahan once asked, "What is the one thing you should do in the first half hour of the day?" The answer is NOTHING, and that is how I begin every day. And by "nothing," I mean that I am spending time with myself. During that time of nothingness, I am breathing of course! I breathe air into my body and then release the breath slowly. With my eyes closed, I relax and wait for the gold glow that appears in the middle of my forehead, right between my eyes. Sometimes it begins as a white or blue dot, and I wait for it to turn golden. I just relax and experience the feeling. When thoughts enter, I look at them as if they are light, fluffy clouds passing overhead. They come and they go; I do not detain them. Sometimes, when I am mediating, it seems like I have been there for hours, and at other times, it seems like only a few moments. The trick to meditating is not to have any tricks! Just remain in the moment and take what you get.

By being present, you may be surprised at what comes up. It's important not to judge but to simply be mindful of your presence and the things around you. Dogs barking, birds singing, bells chiming, passing traffic, children laughing in the street; life is going on around you, so just be mindful of your existence. I like to think that every moment of mediation is extending my life!

In whatever form it takes, meditation is a way for everybody to improve their lives, and for golfers it is a great way to improve your game.

Stress reduction.

When one is relaxed and centered, one can become more focused. The more we meditate, the more we train our bodies and minds to release stress in difficult situations. Reducing stress leads to a growth in self-confidence, positivity, and concentration.

Emotional control.

There are many studies that have shown that a mindful person (someone able to stay in the moment) is better able to control their emotions and moods, which can make the game of golf and life much more pleasurable. The Buddha said, "Stay in the middle of the boat," meaning we should keep our emotions in balance.

Focus.

Most people think too much about the past and the future, ignoring the present. Meditation helps the golfer learn how to stay focused on the task at hand, such as the next tee shot or a long putt. It's important to let go of the last shot and move on to the next without self-judgment of your skills.

Endurance.

Yoga meditation help you keep your body in shape as well as your mind. On average, a golfer walks between 10,000 and 15,000 steps each game, and if the weather or course conditions are difficult, the game can be even tougher. The mind is a muscle that can be strengthened by regular meditation, and that mental strength can support your physical strength, helping you go the distance around the most challenging golf course.

Rest.

Meditation is a natural sleep aid. But an uninterrupted night's sleep can be a rarity for most people because as soon as we close our eyes, our mind runs through everything that has happened that day. If we've had enough peaceful sleep, we are more alert and better able to focus on the golf course.

Healing.

Many sports trainers and managers use meditation as a means of helping athletes prepare to perform, but many studies show that meditation also supports faster healing from injury. Meditation helps rebuild energy (and promotes better sleep, which is needed for healing).

Phil Jackson is one of the most successful NBA coaches of all time, and between 1989 and 2010, he helped the LA Lakers win eleven championships and the New York Knicks win two. He is also called the Zen Master, and in his book, *Sacred Hoops: Spiritual Lessons of a Hardwood Warrior,* he talks about how he used meditation with his athletes:

- To show the power of visualization (the ability to see the ball going through the hoop prior to making the shot, for example.
- To supercharge player's bodies and minds.
- To enable players to come out of their comfort zones.
- To encourage unity within the team (building team spirit, compassion, and understanding).
- To help players find an inner peace.

Meditation Exercises for Golfers

I once played golf with a friend at a course in Texas. We came to a water hole that we had to get over in order to reach the green. He hit his ball—a brand new one—first, and it landed in the water. He hit a second ball—again a brand new one—and got the same result. He tried again and again. A total of seven balls went into the lake. I told him we should move on, but he said, "I am not leaving until I make this shot." I said, "At least use an old ball!" To which he replied, "I have never had an old ball." That is a sign of poor focus.

These exercises can help you "stay in the middle of the boat" as the Buddha advised, remaining emotionally balanced in your life and your game.

Exercise 1: Mindful Visualization

This exercise is a combination of mindful and guided visualization meditation, which I hope will help you improve your game if you practice it often enough.

- Find a quiet place to relax and close out the world for as long as you like.
- Sit in a comfortable position with your back resting against firm support.
- Place your feet flat on the floor with your hands resting in your lap, palms facing towards the sky.
- Sit for few moments doing nothing, letting your body completely relax and keeping your mind clear.
- Simply allow all thoughts to come and go like clouds moving across the sky.
- When you feel relaxed and comfortable, inhale through your nose deeply and hold the breath for a few seconds.
- Exhale through your mouth and feel the breath as it is released from deep within you.

- Inhale and exhale this way repeatedly, feeling the coolness of the air you breathe in and the warmth of the air you breathe out letting go of more tension with each exhalation.
- Now think about the best round of golf you have ever played or your idea of a perfect round.
- Replay that round in your mind.
- If your mind strays, notice that it strayed and then return to the round.
- Think about each effortless swing, and follow the ball as it rises from the tee, performs a perfect arc, and falls on the best place on the fairway.
- Envision your second shot and see how the ball lands perfectly on the green, then picture the flawless putt.
- Picture all your shots like this; away from the hazards of the course.
- When your perfect round replay is over, bring your attention back to your breath (deep inhale and exhale).
- Keeping your eyes closed, raise your arms above your head.
- After a few seconds, open your eyes, bring your hands into your lap, and re-enter reality.

Exercise 2: Grounding

"I love the game so much that I sometimes forget to play it as well as I can. When the first warm sun presses down on your shoulders, when the grass has been mowed for the first time and sits there damp and green, its fresh-cut smell floating up to your nostrils, the sky is deep blue, and an occasional cloud drifts by so white that it dazzles your eyes. A golf course is an intoxicating place."
—Arnold Palmer, from *My Game and Yours*

Every golfer knows the feeling of standing at the tee, surveying the fairway, and experiencing the beauty of the nature all around: green grass and trees, blue water, white clouds, rabbits on the fairway, hawks in the sky, and perhaps a deer or two. Years ago, I played a golf course in northern California near a game reserve. A bobcat showed up and followed us for four holes. It was a great experience! Also, while playing a course in Long Beach, California, a coyote and three pups walked across the fairway in front of us. This connection with the natural environment can lead to the dissolution of the self and integration with Earth: This feeling is "grounding."

Try feeling grounded for yourself through walking in nature. If done at the same time each day, it will not only improve your physical conditioning, it will also improve your emotional well-being. The purpose of this mediation is also to connect to you to the world around you (mindfulness). It is a time to be alone with just you and your thoughts.

Take a walk as short or as long as you like. Be mindful of each step you take, each breath you inhale and exhale. Feel the ground under your feet, the sun and wind on your face, the trees, and the flowers. Let all the things that have happened during the day melt away. If you are walking on the golf course, make a conscious effort to feel the way the grass gives beneath your feet, or feel the grains of sand in the sand trap. Breathe in the fresh air and appreciate the scent of the cut grass.

Although your ball may not have landed where you wanted, focusing on your relationship to the natural features of the course will stop you focusing on your frustration.

Exercise 3: Sleep Like a Rock

This technique will help you get a better night's sleep before game day. When you're lying in bed, preparing to sleep, create a big box in your mind. One by one, picture all the frustrations of the day being placed into the box. This imaginary box will help you let go of things that might keep you awake. At the end of the meditation, imagine locking the box and putting it into the closet.

Once you have locked the box away, it's time to focus on yourself. This exercise takes practice, but if you make it a habit, you will soon master it.

- Lie in your bed in Corpse Pose. Some people like to play soft music (something mellow and instrumental is best).
- Start by deliberately relaxing every part of your head (forehead, space between the eyes, eyelids, lips, and even your ears!). Make sure your teeth are unclenched and your tongue is soft and not pressed against the roof of your mouth.
- When your face is relaxed, focus on your breathing. Inhale and exhale slowly, evenly, and deeply. Your body should now feel heavy.
- Then focus on your toes. Wiggle them then let them relax.
- Working your way up your body, focus on each muscle. Clench each muscle, holding the clench for a few seconds and releasing the tension.
- Pay special attention to the abdomen and shoulders, which is where we hold a lot of tension without realizing it.
- Move all the way up the body back to the head, and imagine all the energy in your body being released through the crown of your head.
- If you haven't already fallen asleep, keep focused on your breathing until you do.

Exercise 4: Meditation on Gratitude

I think we can probably all agree that we tend to take our lives for granted and complain about too many things in our lives. I believe part of the problem is that we see ourselves as separate from the world around us. If we stopped for a moment to appreciate that we are all connected to the world and to each other, we would be far more content.

When things seem to be going wrong in our lives, it is really important to focus on the things that are going right and be grateful for them. When you hit a bad shot, think of the other good ones you hit that day. It is difficult to focus on the next shot if you are focusing on the last one you hit. This is mindfulness.

The Buddha teaches us to be grateful. Period. Gratitude is a mindset that should not be dependent on your social, economic, or physical condition, or social station. This is something I learned while growing up in the South in a very poor family. When I occasionally asked for something that my family could not afford, my mother would say, "Be grateful for what you have, that is your blessing." As a child, it was difficult to understand how I could be grateful. However, throughout my life I have learned to be grateful for everything—even failure. Because I learned valuable lessons through failure, I gained insight into how to use failure to improve my relationships, work, and my life as a whole.

Some people keep a diary of gratefulness. Others, like myself, take time daily to be grateful for all the people in my life who are there for me and for all the blessings I have in my life.

I don't have a one-size-fits-all mediation practice, but if there is just one thing I would urge you all to do is to take time out each day, perhaps several times a day, to close your eyes and say thank you to whatever deity or universal force you believe in. With genuine and unconditional gratitude comes joy and peace, which can see you through the toughest of golf game and difficult periods of your life!

Yoga and meditation has been a way for me to harmonize my mind, body, and spirit. It has also shown me how to practice kindness towards others and myself. I read once that the Buddha would end a meditation or a teaching session with the words that I would now like to leave with you as you close this book:

"May it be of benefit."

Yogi Time

By Victor Stringer

Deep in a forest, high on a hill,
I sat on a rock becoming very still,
In a yogi crossed-legged lotus position;
Finding peace from within was my mission.
As I concentrated on my breathing—
Breathing out to release negative feeling,
Breathing in to enjoy all that lay before me—
I wanted to surrender myself to my senses,
Try to relax and release all of my defenses.
The yogi said, "Meditation should not be used to
Accept; it should be undertaken to become more
Aware of your place in the universe."
As I relaxed, I was overcome with the smells and sounds
Of nature's never-ending splendor around me.
I could hear baby birds chirping in a tree,
And, off in the distance, the sound of a coyote's cry;
Overhead, a gaggle of geese flew by.
I felt the spray of the waterfall just behind me.
The smell of honeysuckle filled the air.
I was no longer aware if it were night or day;
What did it matter anyway? I was on my way!
Back to where I have been many times before.

As I descended further into myself,
I felt as if I were a cloud flowing high in the sky.
I surrendered to the moment, willing to just let things be,
And a great wave of emotion floated through me.
I was aware of a presence enveloping me!
Chills ran from my head down to my feet and back up again;
A bright light seemed to cover me from head to toe.
I knew in my heart I had arrived; there was nowhere else to go!

A peace that I have never known seemed to take control;
All my fears were left behind.
And when once I had been blind;
Now I could see!
From all my illusions I had been set free.
In this moment of awareness, I knew that I could never
Return to the life I had known.
After all, He had allowed me to sit down near His Thrown.
His hand touched the top of my head as He said,
"You have lots of work left to be done.
When it is complete, I will bring you back home.
I will remain in your heart and
Will be there whenever you need me.
I live in your heart. That is my home."
As I awoke from my meditation, I had a feeling I was not alone.
I knew that I would go to that place
Again, as I had done so many times before.
I also know, God, that each time I do, I will
Grow stronger in spirit and get closer to You!

RESOURCES

Inspirational Golf Books

1. *My Game and Yours,* Arnold Palmer, Corgi, 1969.
2. *Darwin on the Green*, Bernard Darwin, Souvenir Press, 1986.
3. *If You Play Golf, You're My Friend*, Harvey Penick, Simon & Shuster, 1993.
4. *What You Know Can Hurt You*, Kip Puterbaugh, Lowell Publishing, 2002.
5. *Golf Tales Through the Eyes of a Caddie*, Aggie Cross, 2010.

Informative Yoga Books

1. *The Yoga Tradition: Its History, Literature, Philosophy and Practice,* Georg Feuerstein, Ph.D. Hohm Press, 2001.
2. *Kundalini Yoga: The Flow of Eternal Power,* Yogi Bhajan, Ph.D., TarcherPerigee, 1998.
3. *YOGA: The Path to Holistic Health,* B.K.S. Iyengar, DK, Revised Edition, 2013.
4. *Anatomy of Fitness: Yoga, the Trainer's Inside Guide to Your Workout,* Goldie Karpel, Hinkler Books, 2014.
5. *Kundalini Yoga: Guidelines for Sadhana (Daily Practice),* Gurucharan Singh Khalsa, Ph.D., Kundalini Research Institute, 2nd edition, 2007.
6. *Meditation for Life,* Martine Batchelor, Wisdom Publications, 2001.

7. *Healing with Ki-Kou: The Secrets of Ancient Chinese Breathing Techniques*, Li Xiuling, Agora Health Books, Second Edition, 2003.

8. *Tantra: The Path of Ecstasy*, Georg Feuerstein, Shambhala,1998.

9. *The Master's Touch: On Being a Sacred Teacher for the New Age*, Yogi Bhajan, Ph.D., Kundalini Research Institute, 1997.

10. *Yoga Body: The Origins of Modern Posture Practice*, Mark Singleton, Oxford University Press, 2010.

11. *Samana,* Luangta Maha Boowa, Forest Dhamma Books, 2011.

Websites

www.yogajournal.com - Includes good descriptions of all the yoga poses and their benefits.

www.18birdies.com - A website that includes yoga exercises for golfers.

www.isha.sadhguru.org - A website about Upa Yoga.

www.lionsroar.com - Buddhist wisdom website.

www.titleist.com - Golf attire and equipment company that also offers seminars and trainings.

www.ingramcontent.com/pod-product-compliance
Lightning Source LLC
Chambersburg PA
CBHW050656270326
41927CB00012B/3050